Asthma Management Module

Ambulatory Care

CLINICAL SKILLS PROGRAM

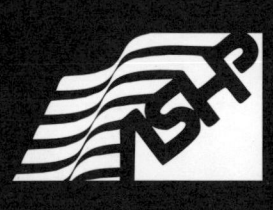

American Society of Health-System Pharmacists

Any correspondence regarding this publication should be sent to the publisher, American Society of Health-System Pharmacists, 7272 Wisconsin Avenue, Bethesda, MD 20814, attn: Cynthia Reilly, Pharmacist Editor/Project Manager, Special Publishing. Produced in conjunction with the ASHP Publications Production Center (Bill Fogle, Technical Editor). Cover and page design by David Wade.

The information presented herein reflects the opinions of the contributors and reviewers. It should not be interpreted as an official policy of ASHP or as an endorsement of any product.

Drug information and its applications are constantly evolving because of ongoing research and clinical experience and are often subject to professional judgment and interpretation by the practitioner and to the uniqueness of a clinical situation. The author and ASHP have made every effort to ensure the accuracy and completeness of the information presented in this book. However, the reader is advised that the publisher, author, contributors, editors, and reviewers cannot be responsible for the continued currency of the information, for any errors or omissions, and/or for any consequences arising from the use of the information in the clinical setting.

The reader is cautioned that ASHP makes no representation, guarantee, or warranty, express or implied, that the use of the information contained in this book will prevent problems with insurers and will bear no responsibility or liability for the results or consequences of its use.

©2000, American Society of Health-System Pharmacists, Inc. All rights reserved.

No part of this publication may be reproduced or transmitted in any form or by any means, electronic or mechanical, including photocopying, microfilming, and recording, or by any information storage and retrieval system, without written permission from the American Society of Health-System Pharmacists. Single copies of the forms may be copied for instructional use only. The forms may not be used or reproduced by any third parties for any commercial purpose. Forms may be modified to meet the special needs of a particular care setting. However, all modified or reproduced forms must acknowledge ASHP as the author and copyright owner (e.g., "Modified from *Ambulatory Care Clinical Skills Program: Asthma Management Module*, American Society of Health-System Pharmacists, Bethesda, Maryland, ©2000. All rights reserved.").

ASHP® is a service mark of the American Society of Health-System Pharmacists, Inc.; registered in the U.S. Patent and Trademark Office.

ISBN: 1-879907-94-1

Contents

Preface iv
Writers and Contributors v
Pharmacy Continuing Education Program and Copyright Information vi
Introduction vii
Asthma Self-Assessment Test ix

Part I: Collecting and Organizing Patient-Specific Information for Patients with Asthma

    *Unit 1: Establishing a Collaborative Relationship with Ambulatory
Asthma Patients* 3

    *Unit 2: Creating a Patient-Specific Database, Part 1: Specific Physical
Assessment Skills* 17

    Unit 3: Creating a Patient-Specific Database, Part 2: Laboratory Data 35

    Unit 4: Creating a Patient-Specific Database, Part 3: Generating the Database .. 43

Part II: Developing an Ambulatory Pharmacist's Care Plan for Patients with Asthma

    *Unit 5: Assessing Current Medication Therapy and Creating a
Therapy Problem List* 99

    Unit 6: Considering the Big Picture: Health Care Needs, Triage, and Referral .. 165

    *Unit 7: Identifying Pharmacotherapeutic and Related Health Care
Goals for Asthma Patients* 179

    Unit 8: Designing a Therapy Regimen for Patients with Asthma 197

    Unit 9: Designing a Monitoring Plan for Patients with Asthma 235

Part III: Managing an Ambulatory Pharmacist's Care Plan for Patients with Asthma

    Unit 10: Implementing a Pharmacist's Care Plan for Patients with Asthma 259

    Unit 11: Evaluating Outcomes for Patients with Asthma 269

    Unit 12: Redesigning the Pharmacist's Care Plan for Patients with Asthma 285

Preface

Pharmacists practicing in ambulatory care settings are increasingly responsible for designing, recommending, and managing patient-specific pharmacotherapy regimens. Asthma is a prevalent chronic disease that is highly amenable to pharmacist involvement. The ambulatory care pharmacist works with the patient in designing a plan of care to optimize asthma-related health outcomes.

The *Ambulatory Care Clinical Skills Program: Asthma Management Module* builds on and applies the skills learned in the *Ambulatory Care Clinical Skills Program: Core Module*. Pharmacists will work with asthma patients to generate a database, assess the patient's therapy, identify health care needs, identify pharmacotherapeutic and related health care goals, recommend a therapeutic plan, evaluate outcomes, and redesign plans as needed. Upon completion of this module, ambulatory care pharmacists will be well prepared to take their place on the health care team, working with asthma patients.

Pharmacists who complete the *Core Module* as well as this module will find the information essential to the development or enhancement of asthma care practice. This module is designed to apply the information from the *Core Module* to the care of a patient with asthma. Unit 1 will address why and how you should develop collaborative relationships with patients with asthma. Units 2, 3, and 4 will teach you how to create a patient-specific database. You will learn to assess medications and create a drug therapy problem list in unit 5; the importance of considering the overall patient health care needs, triage, and referral in unit 6; and identifying health care goals in unit 7. The design of a therapy regimen for a patient with asthma will be discussed in unit 8. Units 9 through 12 will focus on the development, monitoring, implementation, and reassessment of the care plan for a patient with asthma.

Finally, this module offers American Council on Pharmaceutical Education (ACPE)–approved continuing education (CE) credit to those students who successfully pass the CE tests. Directions for those tests are enclosed with this module.

Writers

Charlotte Anne Kenreigh, Pharm.D.

Linda Timm Wagner, Pharm.D.

Contributors

ASHP wishes to acknowledge the following people who contributed their time and expertise to the development of this text:

Reza Ally
John A. Armistead
J. Lynn Bass
Nick P. Beckey
Darrel Bjornson
Carrie Bocckelman
Irene Contreras
Leslie Dotson Jaggers
George J. Dydek
Tammy S. Ellickson
Nancy T. Fong
Tom Frank
Jon J. Glover
William Griffin
Phillip Jennings
H. William Kelly
Kristine E. Keplar

Lisa B. Korman
Lynnae M. Mahaney
Patricia Marshik
Susan J. Morikawa
Coleen Nelson
Sandra Oh Clarke
Lisa Oliver
Patricia Powers
Cynthia Reilly
Jane S. Ricciuti
Naomi Schultheis
Marie A. Smith
Suellyn J. Sorenson
Teresa L. Wild
Helen Yee
Mary H. Zimmerman

Pharmacy Continuing Education Program

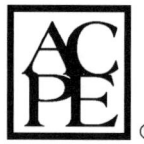

By successfully completing the three continuing education tests for the *Ambulatory Care Clinical Skills Program: Asthma Management Module*, you can earn 0.9 continuing education units (CEUs). The American Council on Pharmaceutical Education (ACPE) numbers for the *Ambulatory Care Clinical Skills Program: Asthma Management Module* are Part I: Collecting and Organizing Patient-Specific Information for Patients with Asthma, 204-000-99-051-H01; Part II: Developing an Ambulatory Pharmacist's Care Plan for Patients with Asthma, 204-000-99-052-H01; Part III: Managing an Ambulatory Pharmacist's Care Plan for Patients with Asthma 204-000-99-053-H01. The tests and answer sheets are bound separately from this book.

The American Society of Health-System Pharmacists is approved by the ACPE as a provider of continuing pharmaceutical education.

Copyright Information

Single copies of the blank forms contained in this book may be distributed to individual students of the Ambulatory Care Clinical Skills Program at no charge and for educational purposes only. The forms may not be reproduced by third parties for commercial purposes. Forms may be modified to meet the special needs of a particular education program. However, all modified documents must acknowledge ASHP as the author and copyright owner (e.g., "Modified from *Ambulatory Care Clinical Skills Program: Asthma Management Module*, American Society of Health-System Pharmacists, Bethesda, Maryland, ©2000. All rights reserved.").

Introduction

Who Can Benefit From Using the *Ambulatory Care Clinical Skills Program: Asthma Management Module*

ASHP created the *Ambulatory Care Clinical Skills Program: Asthma Management Module* as part of a profession-wide effort to increase pharmacy's involvement in clinical practice and pharmaceutical care in the ambulatory care setting. Both pharmacists and pharmacy students can enhance their clinical skills by engaging in these self-study activities. Current staff pharmacists, pharmacists in the midst of a career change, recent graduates wishing to sharpen their skills, and pharmacy students involved in clinical clerkships can benefit from this program, working alone or as part of a staff development program.

The skills referred to in the title are problem-solving skills. Before you can begin to solve a problem, however, you must have content knowledge related to the problem area. To achieve the objectives of the *Asthma Management Module*, you should have a solid foundation in the following knowledge areas related to asthma:
- pathophysiology
- clinical pharmacology and therapeutics
- clinical laboratory data interpretation
- clinical pharmacokinetics
- medical terminology and abbreviations

The *Asthma Management Module* presumes the participants have current mastery of these areas and makes no effort to reteach pharmacy school didactics. Instead, this module helps you apply these pharmacy knowledge areas in solving asthma drug therapy problems. Participants should take the self-assessment test found on pages ix–xv, prior to beginning work on this module. A score of less than 90% indicates that the participant requires additional didactic preparation prior to beginning coursework. Your self-assessment test results will also demonstrate specific areas where reinforcement of content is required.

What To Do If You Need Didactic Preparation

You may feel uneasy about your didactic preparation for this module. Perhaps it has been some time since you were a pharmacy student and your didactic preparation is outdated, maybe you went to a pharmacy school that did not emphasize one of the content areas required by the *Asthma Management Module*. Or perhaps your job has been focused on distribution, so you are rusty on therapeutic concepts. If so, use the clinical library noted below to refresh or enhance your knowledge. Your colleagues in pharmacy are also potential sources of help. Your department director, clinical coordinator, staff development coordinator, or professor at the local college of pharmacy may assist you in developing a plan of reading assignments.

The preface to the *Core Module* text lists several recommended references to develop your library. These include basic medical texts, physical assessment texts, pharmacotherapeutic texts, pharmacokinetic application texts, and other valuable resources.

There are additional references specific to asthma that you may find useful in working through this module and in future practice. Several recommendations include:

1. National Asthma Education and Prevention Program. Guidelines for the Diagnosis and Management of Asthma, Expert Panel Report 2. NIH Publication No. 97-4051. Also available electronically at http://www.nhlbi.nih.gov/guidelines/asthma/asthgdln.htm.

2. Lemanske RF, Green CG. Asthma in infancy and childhood. In: *Allergy Principles & Practice*, *Volume II*. 5th ed. Middleton E, Ellis E, Yuninger JW, et al., editors. St. Louis, MO: Mosby; 1998. p. 877–900.

3. Mathison DA. Asthma in adults. In: *Allergy Principles & Practice*, *Volume II*. 5th ed. Middleton E, Ellis E, Yuninger JW, et al., editors. St. Louis, MO: Mosby; 1998. p. 901–26.

How This Program Is Organized

The *Asthma Management Module* is organized into twelve units. Building on the skills learned in the *Core Module*, you will design, recommend, and manage asthma-specific pharmacotherapeutic plans.

The Best Way to Use the Clinical Skills Program

When using the *Asthma Management Module*, you can work either alone or as part of a group. If you are working alone, you may want to ask your practice site supervisor to help you practice the clinical skills you are learning. To gain competence in assessment of physical parameters, you must participate in an educational environment that includes repetitive hands-on demonstration and practice with trained educators.

The units of the *Asthma Management Module* should be studied in sequential order. The module is a carefully structured, systematic approach to acquiring drug therapy and drug information problem-solving skills.

Self-Assessment Questions

1. Circle all of the following that are signs or symptoms of asthma.
   A. wheezing
   B. cough
   C. sore throat
   D. weight loss
   E. dermatitis
   F. difficulty sleeping
   G. exercise intolerance

2. Which of the following is the primary cause of wheezing?
   A. Inflammatory response results in bronchoconstriction.
   B. Environmental trigger directly stimulates bronchoconstriction.
   C. Poor airway compliance causes bronchoconstriction.
   D. Increased mucus secretions plug airways.

3. Which of the following is the primary cause of nighttime cough?
   A. excessive corticosteroid use during daytime hours
   B. excessive beta-adrenergic agonist use during daytime hours
   C. increased concentrations of mold in nighttime air
   D. decreased endogenous cortisol levels

4. Which of the following best estimates the number of people in the United States with asthma?
   A. 2 million
   B. 8 million
   C. 15 million
   D. 30 million

5. Which of the following best describes the incidence of asthma?
   A. It is significantly increasing.
   B. It is slowly increasing.
   C. It is decreasing.
   D. The incidence is relatively stable.

6. Mortality associated with asthma is most prevalent in which population?
   A. pediatric
   B. geriatric
   C. African Americans
   D. the mortality rate is similar in all populations

7. Circle all of the following that are risk factors for asthma.
   A. nasal polyps
   B. aspirin allergy
   C. atopy
   D. vegetarian diet
   E. gastroesophageal reflux
   F. chronic sinusitis
   G. alopecia
   H. rheumatoid arthritis
   I. history of early life injury to the airways (bronchopulmonary dysplasia or pneumonia)

8. Which of the following are considered triggers for patients with asthma?
   A. exercise
   B. respiratory infections
   C. allergic responses
   D. menstrual cycle
   E. bright sunshine
   F. cold temperatures
   G. smoke
   H. emotions
   I. diet
   J. caffeinated beverages
   K. alcohol

9. Fluctuations of the endogenous concentration of which of the following hormones could trigger an asthma exacerbation?
   A. estrogen
   B. cortisol
   C. somatropin
   D. insulin
   E. growth factor
   F. gastrin

10. Which of the following best describes the pathogenesis of asthma?
    A. marked hypertrophy and hyperplasia of airway smooth muscle
    B. decreased lung elasticity
    C. increased white blood cells in lungs
    D. alpha-1 antitrypsin deficiency

11. Which of the following best describes the pathogenesis of asthma?
    A. inflammatory cell infiltration of the airways
    B. decreased beta-receptors in the airways
    C. bacterial colonization
    D. mucus plugging secondary to altered sodium channels

12. Which of the following best describes the pathogenesis of asthma?
    A. Direct stimulation of beta-receptors results in bronchospasm.
    B. Inflammatory mediators are activated and result in bronchial hyperreactivity.
    C. Cyclooxygenase stimulation releases platelet-activating factor.
    D. Acetylcholinesterase stimulation results in bronchial hyperreactivity.

13. Which of the following best characterizes mild-intermittent asthma?
    A. symptoms ≤2 times per week
    B. mild daily symptoms
    C. frequent exacerbations
    D. need for daily inhaled corticosteroid therapy

14. Which of the following best characterizes moderate-persistent asthma?
    A. daily symptoms with weekly nighttime symptoms
    B. continual symptoms
    C. normal PEF
    D. symptoms that limit physical activity

15. Which of the following best characterizes severe-persistent asthma?
    A. continual symptoms with frequent nighttime symptoms
    B. daily use of inhaled short-acting beta-adrenergic agonist
    C. PEF 80% of predicted
    D. brief exacerbations varying in intensity

16. Which of the following best explains the clinical course of asthma?
    A. Patients begin with mild persistent asthma and progress over time.
    B. Patients with severe-persistent asthma never improve.
    C. Mild-intermittent asthma progresses to moderate asthma in 50% of patients.
    D. Patients may fluctuate between severity levels of asthma over time.

17. Which of the following best explains the clinical course of asthma?
    A. Asthma symptoms are consistent day and night in most patients.
    B. Symptoms always occur immediately postexposure to a trigger.
    C. Some patients experience improvement in asthma symptoms during pregnancy.
    D. Patients that experience only nighttime symptoms do not need prophylactic therapy.

18. Which of the following best explains the clinical course of asthma?
    A. Patients may not recognize the severity of symptoms.
    B. Patients are acutely aware of the severity of symptoms.
    C. The majority of pediatric patients with asthma outgrow their disease.
    D. Patients with asthma must limit their physical activity.

19. Circle all of the following that describe an accepted treatment for asthma.
    A. theophylline
    B. ipratropium
    C. calcium supplements
    D. echinacea
    E. prednisone
    F. terbutaline
    G. maprotiline
    H. Primatene Mist

20. Which of the following best describes why an inhaled corticosteroid is an effective treatment for asthma?
    A. produces bronchodilation
    B. blocks beta receptors
    C. reduces airway inflammation
    D. stimulates alpha receptors

21. Which of the following best describes why an inhaled beta-adrenergic agonist is an effective treatment for asthma?
    A. reduces airway inflammation
    B. relieves acute bronchoconstriction
    C. blocks beta receptors
    D. upregulates beta receptors

22. Circle all of the following that are indications for the use of salmeterol.
    A. improvement of exercise tolerance
    B. as rescue therapy
    C. for mild-intermittent asthma
    D. for nocturnal asthma
    E. for pregnancy-induced asthma

23. Which of the following best explains why persistent asthma is an indication for corticosteroids?
    A. These are the only drugs that work in long-term management of asthma.
    B. The mechanism of action of these drugs is targeted at the underlying cause of asthma.
    C. There are no side effects when these medications are inhaled.
    D. These are the least expensive therapies available.

24. Which of the following best explains why mild-intermittent asthma is an indication for beta-adrenergic agonist therapies?
    A. prevent exacerbations when used on a scheduled basis
    B. prevent airway inflammation in patients with mild disease
    C. treat the symptoms of occasional exacerbations in patients with mild disease
    D. relatively nontoxic and easy to use

25. Circle all of the following that are contraindications for the use of zileuton in the treatment of asthma?
    A. liver disease
    B. renal disease
    C. age <18
    D. severe-persistent asthma
    E. moderate-persistent asthma
    F. aspirin sensitivity
    G. relief of acute symptoms

26. Which of the following best explains why an underlying seizure disorder not treated with anticonvulsants is a contraindication to theophylline?
    A. theophylline lowers the seizure threshold
    B. theophylline raises the seizure threshold
    C. theophylline causes pseudo-seizures
    D. theophylline interferes with GABA

27. Which of the following best explains the mechanism of action of zafirlukast?
    A. directly stimulates bronchial smooth muscle to produce bronchodilation
    B. stimulates beta receptors to produce bronchodilation
    C. antagonizes leukotriene receptors; therefore, interfering with the inflammatory process
    D. increases cGMP to produce bronchodilation

28. Which of the following best describes the mechanism of action of salmeterol?
    A. directly stimulates bronchial smooth muscle to produce bronchodilation
    B. increases beta receptors to produce bronchodilation
    C. antagonizes leukotriene receptors; therefore, interfering with the inflammatory process
    D. stimulates cGMP to produce bronchodilation

29. Which of the following best describes the mechanism of action of ipratropium?
    A. directly stimulates bronchial smooth muscle to produce bronchodilation
    B. stimulates beta receptors to produce bronchodilation
    C. antagonizes leukotriene receptors; therefore, interfering with the inflammatory process
    D. increases cGMP to produce bronchodilation

30. Which of the following best explains the pharmacokinetics of theophylline?
    A. It is 100% bioavailable.
    B. It is highly protein bound.
    C. It is ineffective at serum concentrations <10 mg/L.
    D. It has a narrow therapeutic range.

31. Which of the following best explains the pharmacokinetics of theophylline?
    A. linear
    B. nonlinear
    C. chiou
    D. linear over therapeutic range, nonlinear at higher concentrations

32. Which of the following best describes the pharmacokinetics of zafirlukast?
    A. immediate onset
    B. rapidly absorbed
    C. predominantly renally eliminated
    D. highly protein bound

33. Which of the following best describes a treatment regimen for a patient with asthma?
    A. Serevent 2 puffs two times daily, albuterol 2 puffs as needed for increased symptoms
    B. Serevent 2 puffs two times daily, Intal 2 puffs as needed for increased symptoms
    C. Intal 2 puffs as needed for increased symptoms
    D. Serevent 2 puffs as needed for increased symptoms

34. Which of the following best describes a treatment regimen for a pediatric patient with asthma?
    A. Albuterol syrup 5 cc three times daily
    B. Intal nebulizer solution 2 cc four times daily with Ventolin nebulizer solution 0.3 cc four times daily
    C. Intal nebulizer solution 2 cc four times daily, Ventolin nebulizer solution 0.3 cc as needed for increased symptoms
    D. Azmacort nebulizer solution 2 cc four times daily with Ventolin nebulizer solution 0.3 cc four times daily

35. Which of the following best describes a treatment regimen for a patient with nocturnal cough from asthma?
    A. Robitussin with codeine 10 ml as needed for nighttime cough
    B. Guiatuss 15 ml as needed for nighttime cough
    C. Albuterol syrup 10 ml as needed for nighttime cough
    D. Serevent inhaler 2 puffs at bedtime

36. Which of the following describes a drug-drug interaction in a patient treated for asthma?
    A. theophylline-Azmacort
    B. theophylline-Tilade
    C. theophylline-Tagamet
    D. theophylline-Intal

37. Which of the following categories is associated with a drug-disease interaction in a patient with asthma?
    A. acetylcholinesterase inhibitors
    B. calcium channel blockers
    C. alpha blockers
    D. beta-adrenergic blockers

38. Which of the following pairs does *not* represent a therapeutic duplication in a patient with asthma?
    A. Serevent-Ventolin
    B. Ventolin-Alupent
    C. Tilade-Intal
    D. Azmacort-Pulmicort

39. Circle all of the following that describe common adverse reactions when treating patients with asthma.
    A. shaking
    B. nausea
    C. fever
    D. increased hemoglobin
    E. increased appetite
    F. oral thrush
    G. vulvovaginal candidiasis
    H. poor sleep quality
    I. somnolence
    J. decreased appetite

40. Which of the following therapies for asthma are reported to leave a bad taste in the patient's mouth?
    A. Intal nebulizer solution
    B. Intal oral inhaler
    C. Alupent oral inhaler
    D. Tilade oral inhaler

41. Which of the following best explains the difference between side effects of oral corticosteroids and inhaled corticosteroids?
    A. Oral corticosteroids are different biochemically from inhaled steroids.
    B. Inhaled corticosteroids are not absorbed.
    C. Absorption from inhaled doses leads to lower systemic blood levels.
    D. Absorption from inhaled doses leads to higher systemic blood levels.

42. The addition of a controller medication to the medication regimen for a patient with persistent asthma _____.
    A. increases medication costs unnecessarily
    B. decreases overall medication costs
    C. increases medication costs and decreases overall health care costs
    D. decreases medication costs and increases overall health care costs

43. A patient being started on a corticosteroid inhaler should expect to get sustained benefit _____.
    A. immediately
    B. within 1 or 2 weeks
    C. after 2 months
    D. within 1 or 2 days

44. The underlying causative factor for asthma is _____.
    A. genetic
    B. not fully known
    C. slowed lung maturation
    D. overproduction of histamine

Self-Assessment Answers

1. A, B, F, G
2. A
3. D
4. C
5. A
6. C
7. A, B, C, E, F, I
8. A, B, C, D, F, G, H
9. A, B
10. A
11. A
12. B
13. A
14. A
15. A
16. D
17. C
18. A
19. A, B, E, F
20. C
21. B
22. A, D
23. B
24. C
25. A, D, E
26. A
27. C
28. A
29. D
30. D
31. D
32. B
33. A
34. C
35. D
36. C
37. D
38. A
39. A, B, E, F, H
40. D
41. C
42. C
43. B
44. B

Part I

Collecting and Organizing Patient-Specific Information for Patients with Asthma

Establishing a Collaborative Relationship with Ambulatory Asthma Patients

UNIT 1

Unit Objectives	4
Unit Organization	4
Asthma: Disease Influences on Pharmacist-Patient Relationships	4
Patient Emotional and Physical Characteristics Affecting Establishment of a Collaborative Relationship	5
Patient Empowerment	5
Pediatric Patients	5
Patient Health Care Beliefs	7
Example Case	7
Adult Patients	8
Assessing Asthma Triggers	8
Opportunities for Collaborative Practice in the Management of Asthma	9
Establishing a Professional Relationship	10
Case Study	11
Practice Example	12
Summary	13
References	13
Self-Study Questions	14
Self-Study Answers	15

Patients with chronic diseases, such as asthma, can benefit from the establishment of a long-term relationship with their pharmacist. With the emphasis on ambulatory care, pharmacists have increased opportunities to actively participate in the management of patients. The chronic nature of asthma makes it possible for a pharmacist to develop an ongoing collaborative partnership with asthma patients. Through this relationship, pharmacists participate in the pharmaceutical care of their patients, ensuring that the patients understand their disease and medication regimen and are achieving desired outcomes of therapy with minimal adverse effects.

The establishment of a collaborative relationship is essential for the management of patients with asthma. As you will learn in units 2 and 3, in contrast to some other chronic diseases, few laboratory tests and simple physical examinations are used to guide asthma therapy. The most important information obtained in asthma management is the patient history. Patients' descriptions of their symptoms over time and their own ability to recognize times of distress are critical in identifying and managing appropriate drug therapy. A collaborative relationship cannot be achieved without a foundation of respect and trust between you and your patient.

Many asthma patients continue to suffer from uncontrolled disease. A large number of people have unrecognized asthma and use over-the-counter remedies for self-treatment of symptoms consistent with asthma. Their pharmacist may be the first health care provider to recognize a lack of asthma control. Education in the technique and role in therapy of prescription medications, the use of nonprescription medications, and the reinforcement and clarification of treatment plans are essential components of asthma management. Pharmacists have the ability to monitor refill histories; evaluate prescription, over-the-counter, and herbal medication use; and provide ongoing education in controlling asthma episodes.

After completing this unit, through discussion and case application, you will gain knowledge and understanding of the skills necessary to help patients with asthma in your practice.

Unit Objectives

After you successfully complete this unit, you will be able to:

- explain disease influences on pharmacist-patient relationships;
- explain the emotional and physical characteristics of ambulatory care patients with asthma that may affect the establishment of a collaborative patient-pharmacist relationship; and
- when given a description of an ambulatory care patient with asthma, design an effective strategy for establishing a collaborative professional relationship with that patient.

Unit Organization

To begin, this unit will discuss asthma and the unique emotional and physical characteristics of a patient with asthma that may affect the development of a professional relationship. Next, the unit will provide strategies for forming a collaborative relationship. Finally, a case study and practice example will be provided to help develop these skills.

Asthma: Disease Influences on Pharmacist-Patient Relationships

Asthma, a chronic respiratory condition, affects approximately 14.6 million Americans. Approximately one third of patients with asthma are children <18 years of age.[1] Asthma has continued to rise significantly in all age groups, including children. It develops most frequently in childhood, although asthma may develop during any period of life. Childhood asthma is most often associated with atopy, viral illness, or allergies. Adult-onset asthma does not have a clear association with allergy. Some adult patients have allergies, whereas other adult patients have asthma associated with nasal polyps and aspirin sensitivity, work-related exposures, or chronic sinusitis. Work-related exposures may be difficult to recognize because symptoms may not begin for several hours following exposure.

Not properly managed and controlled, asthma can be life threatening. The mortality associated with asthma has continued to increase in the past several years. The age-adjusted mortality rate associated with asthma increased 67% between 1979 and 1995.[2] An estimated 5500 deaths each year in the United States are attributed to asthma.[1]

Asthma-related mortality occurs more frequently among African Americans than among white Americans.

The economic impact of asthma is substantial. In 1993, the health care costs of asthma were estimated to be more than $12.5 billion (1993) dollars. This estimate includes direct medical costs and indirect costs associated with loss of productivity from work and school. A large portion of direct health care costs is associated with emergent inpatient admissions from uncontrolled asthma. The largest financial burden associated with asthma can be attributed to 20% of patients diagnosed with asthma.[2]

Airway inflammation and an episodic nature characterize asthma in the majority of patients. Airways become inflamed in response to a variety of stimuli or triggers. Airway inflammation results in variable airflow obstruction characterized by wheezing, breathlessness, chest tightness, and cough (especially at night and in the early morning). Asthma severity varies from mild intermittent to severe persistent. The most recent definitions for the degrees of asthma severity have been outlined in the National Heart, Lung, and Blood Institute Expert Panel Report 2 and are described in **Table 1**.[3]

The severity of a patient's asthma may fluctuate. This fluctuation reflects varying control of inflammatory episodes and may be attributed to seasonal triggers, environmental factors, understanding of the disease, exercise, infections, compliance with medications, and other health conditions.

Patient Emotional and Physical Characteristics Affecting Establishment of a Collaborative Relationship

Patients may experience few or no symptoms for long periods of time and then present with an acute exacerbation. This fluctuation in symptoms may cause patients to downplay the seriousness of the disease. Patients, especially adolescents, tend to become cavalier in their approach to asthma when their symptoms are well controlled. Being different from everyone else is certainly a major concern for anyone with a chronic disease, especially children. Treatment of asthma needs to include a discussion of this emotional component. Patients and caregivers need to be aware of the unique concerns of patients with asthma. Strategies aimed at making the patient feel less different need to be incorporated into the treatment plan. Such strategies may include altering therapy to avoid, whenever possible, the need to use medications in work, social, or school settings. Patients need to be fully aware that allowing an exacerbation to go unchecked may be life threatening. Even patients with mild intermittent disease can develop life-threatening airway obstruction.

People with asthma do not look any different from people without asthma unless they have had chronic exacerbations. Some patients may, on physical examination, present with hyperexpansion of the thorax, or barrel chest. Accessory muscle use may also be noted, especially in pediatric patients. Patients with chronic exacerbations who have poor oxygen exchange may also develop clubbing of the fingers. The presence of nasal polyps and aspirin sensitivity has also been associated with asthma. Another subset of patients with asthma have evidence of atopic dermatitis or eczema. Refer to unit 2 for further discussion of the assessment of a patient's general appearance.

Patient Empowerment

Patients must learn to take an active role in the management of their asthma and prevent and reduce exacerbations by controlling airway inflammation. The National Heart, Lung, and Blood Institute Asthma Education and Prevention Program Expert Panel Report 2 released in 1997 offers national guidelines for the diagnosis and management of asthma.[3] The goal of these guidelines is to encourage the prevention of asthma exacerbations through the prevention of airway inflammation. The role of patients in the treatment and control of the disease is paramount to successful therapy. The chronic nature of asthma means that the majority of asthma care is not provided in an acute care setting. The ambulatory care environment is the ideal setting to support patients with asthma. Patients who receive appropriate information and continued support are more likely to make appropriate treatment and compliance decisions. A patient needs to be an important participant in the design and establishment of a treatment plan. Engaging the patient in the management of the disease will require different approaches, depending on the patient's age.

Pediatric Patients

Health care providers administering to pediatric

Table 1. Classification of Asthma Severity by Clinical Features Before Treatment[a]

	Symptoms[b]	Nighttime Symptoms	Lung Function
STEP 4 *Severe persistent*	Continual symptoms Limited physical activity Frequent exacerbations	Frequent	FEV_1 or PEF ≤60% predicted PEF variability >30%
STEP 3 *Moderate persistent*	Daily symptoms Daily use of inhaled short-acting $beta_2$-adrenergic agonist Exacerbations affect activity Exacerbations ≥2 times/week; may last days	>1 time/week	FEV_1 or PEF >60% or <80% predicted PEF variability >30%
STEP 2 *Mild persistent*	Symptoms >2 times a week but <1 time a day Exacerbations may affect activity	>2 times/month	FEV_1 or PEF ≥80% predicted PEF variability 20–30%
STEP 1 *Mild intermittent*	Symptoms ≤2 times/week Asymptomatic and normal PEF between exacerbations Exacerbations brief (from a few hours to a few days); intensity may vary	≤2 times/month	FEV_1 or PEF ≥80% predicted PEF variability <20%

FEV_1, forced expiratory volume in 1 second; PEF, peak expiratory flow (PEF).

[a]The presence of one of the features of severity is sufficient to place a patient in that category. An individual should be assigned to the most severe grade in which any feature occurs. The characteristics noted in this table are general and may overlap because asthma is highly variable. Furthermore, an individual's classification may change over time.
[b]Patients at any level of severity can have mild, moderate, or severe exacerbations. Some patients with intermittent asthma experience severe and life-threatening exacerbations separated by long periods of normal lung function and no symptoms.

Source: reprinted from reference 3.

patients will need the involvement of the patient's caregiver as well as the patient. Caregivers may include parents, day care providers, coaches, teachers, school nurses, and extracurricular group leaders. Anyone that will be directly responsible for a child will need to be informed about the patient's asthma, medications, and what to do in case of an exacerbation. Younger children will need the caregiver to coordinate and assist in the use and monitoring of medications. It is extremely important that the caregiver understands the treatment plan and is able to act in the best interest of the child.

As children get older, more responsibility can be placed on them. The age that is most appropriate for self-administration of medication will depend on the maturity of the child. Some children may not be prepared to handle the responsibility of taking control of managing their disease until well into their teenage years. Other children as young as 9 or 10 years old may be able to successfully take on this responsibility.

During the pediatric years, it's important to

recognize that the caregiver-child relationship may affect the management of the disease. When children rebel, struggles over the administration of medications may ensue. As children become preteens and teenagers, issues may surface about being different from others because of asthma. Children need to be encouraged to engage in physical activities. In the past, patients with asthma have been stereotyped as physically unfit and not capable of excelling in sports. In fact, many professional athletes have asthma and are able to excel in sports while maintaining control of their disease. Providing pediatric patients with such examples may help them deal with the disease.

The emotional component of this disease may result in the child purposefully exposing him or herself to situations that may trigger an asthma exacerbation. The child may also refuse to take medications when needed in order to seem like one of the crowd. Children may find it embarrassing to use an inhaler, but if they are encouraged to explain the use and need for an inhaler to their friends and teachers ahead of time, the embarrassment may be reduced. Children need to be encouraged to take on the responsibility of asthma management. Other emotional factors may also precipitate an episode of asthma. Emotional stress (including strenuous laughing or crying) and anxiety may trigger an episode.

Peer pressure to be daring, go to parties, and smoke may place the adolescent in a precarious situation. Although such behavior is not characteristic of all adolescent patients, careful attention needs to be given to this potential concern. The health care provider should foster a relationship with patients in this age group. The parent or caregiver remains important for moral support but plays a lesser role in treatment decisions.

Pediatric patients need to be included in discussions about their care and educated about the disease and its management.[4] Adolescent patients, in particular, need to be given the responsibility for the outcome of their disease. Health care professionals cannot expect that a parent or caregiver can simply mandate that a patient take care of him- or herself. Agreement on the treatment plan must be reached by all members of the team, including the patient.

Patient Health Care Beliefs

Education about the long-term effects of medications must be addressed. Concerns about the use of corticosteroids in the pediatric population raises issues not only for parents but for children as well. It is important to assess the patient's and caregiver's understanding of the medication, its use, and any potential long-term complications. Most important, the patient needs to be included in making therapy and personal goals.

Example Case

Let's look at a possible patient-pharmacist encounter. Angel Cordle is a 16-year-old, 150-lb female. She has battled asthma since she was a child and has struggled to be one of the crowd. Her mother comes to your pharmacy to pick up some oral prednisone that Angel needs to control her most recent episode of asthma. Angel is with her mother but doesn't come into the pharmacy. Her mother is obviously distraught and angry with Angel for going out with friends that smoke. Angel's mother wants to know what she should do and asks your advice.

PHARMACIST:
"Angel needs to stay away from people who smoke. The next exacerbation could land her in the hospital, or worse. You need to tell her she can't go to places where people smoke anymore. She'll listen to you, you are her mother, after all."

MRS. CORDLE:
"That's what I've been saying, but I haven't been able to get through to her. She's at that age where she thinks everything I say is wrong and that I'm trying to make her life miserable."

PHARMACIST:
"I can certainly understand your frustration, but you'll have to try and convince her that it is for her own good."

This interaction sets a tone for this and future interactions, and you can see that the tone is negative and accusatory. Communication may be hampered. Let's look at another approach to Angel's case that effectively communicates a plan.

PHARMACIST:
"It's awfully hard for an adolescent to have a chronic disease and still feel normal during this awkward time in life. Peer pressure can be tremendous. Do you think Angel would be interested in setting up a time to come in and discuss her asthma and medications with me? Sometimes things go better if we give her the ability to take on the management and responsibility for her own health."

MRS. CORDLE:
"Well, that sounds like a good idea. Why don't I see if she'll come in and set something up with you now. I just assumed she should know all of the right things to do since she's had asthma for so long, but maybe you will be able to help her. I'll send her in."

Angel comes into the pharmacy looking resentful that her mother has asked her to talk to the pharmacist.

PHARMACIST:
"Hi, Angel. My name is Karen and I'm a pharmacist with a lot of experience talking with teenagers about their asthma. Your mom told me you've had a little bit of trouble with your asthma lately. Do you think you'd like to set up a time to come in and sit down with me to talk about your asthma? We can go back into my office where it will be private."

ANGEL:
"My mother is so hysterical, she exaggerates everything. But I suppose I could come in. Maybe then I can get my mother off my back. She is such a nag!"

PHARMACIST:
"Great, does one day after school next week work for you?"

ANGEL:
"I guess Monday will work, at 3 p.m. Do I need to bring my mom?"

PHARMACIST:
"Monday sounds fine. No, let's make this just between you and me. If you'd like, your mom can come in at the end of our talk and we can review some of the information with her. Don't worry, it won't take long and we'll go over your medications and talk about how they are working for you."

In the latter example, the pharmacist acknowledges that adolescence can be difficult for a patient with asthma and attempts to involve the patient in the discussion. The pharmacist is trying to place Angel in a position of responsibility for her own disease and health outcomes, giving Angel the opportunity to have autonomy. The pharmacist does not try to dictate how Angel should act, offering her instead the opportunity to engage in a discussion about her disease. Using this approach, the pharmacist allows Angel to take an active role in the management of her asthma and assists her in the development of problem-solving skills. Including parents at the end of the session will serve to solidify the supportive role of parents.

Adult Patients

Adults may run into emotional problems associated with asthma as well. Adults, like children, do not want to be singled out as sickly or different. They may avoid using medications when they are needed in order to fit in with everyone else. Workplace situations may not be conducive to administering needed medications. Some workplace environments may actually precipitate occupational asthma. Adult patients must be encouraged to explain asthma and their triggers to employers if necessary. Patients should be cautioned before they approach management with their concerns; in some cases, questions about potential occupational exposures have resulted in employees losing their jobs. Before a patient decides to discuss this health issue with an employer, he or she needs to be aware of the potential ramifications. In most cases, employers will be glad to work with employees to manage the situation; for additional information, refer to the Americans with Disabilities Act federal guidelines. Aside from workplace exposures, adults may find themselves in social situations where tobacco smoke or illicit drug use is present. Adults, like pediatric patients, need to be encouraged to avoid these situations.

The patient's psychological outlook on the disease will ultimately affect the decision to adhere to a prescribed care plan. A patient who views asthma as intermittent episodes rather than a chronic disease will be less likely to comply with preventive therapy. The Health Belief Model describes cost-benefit analysis done by patients to determine whether they feel the need to follow a given treatment plan.[5] Patients who believe their disease is significant and that preventive therapy will be beneficial in the long run without major lifestyle complications will be more apt to follow a treatment plan than patients who do not hold a similar belief.

Assessing Asthma Triggers

Because of the intermittent nature of asthma, patients may not be aware of the importance of maintaining a close, collaborative relationship with a pharmacist and health care team. It is important as a pharmacist to educate patients about the chronic nature of the disease and the need to keep airway inflammation to a minimum even during periods of seemingly inactive disease. Patients need to be aware of situations that may trigger an episode.

When assessing a patient, the diurnal nature of asthma must be considered. Because of the lower endogenous cortisol levels (levels are lowest at 4 a.m.), many patients experience nighttime symptoms, with fewer problems during the daytime. Always ask a patient about the presence of nighttime symptoms. Potential asthma triggers are listed in **Table 2**.[3,6]

Your role as a pharmacist is to not only encourage patients to be aware of the triggers for their disease, but also to help them determine ways to avoid these exposures and to teach them what

Table 2. Asthma Exacerbation Triggers[3, 6]

Viral respiratory infections

Gastroesophageal reflux

Environmental allergens

Animals

Exercise

Occupational chemicals and irritants

Irritants (smoke, dust, and pollution)

Emotional expression

Medications

Food or food additives

Weather/season changes

Endocrine factors (pregnancy, menstruation, and thyroid)

should be done should an exacerbation occur. You need to be involved on a continuing basis to serve as a coach and continue in the development of a patient-pharmacist relationship. Education and reinforcement of proper inhaler technique needs to be offered with every encounter. This reinforcement will encourage patients to self-manage their disease. Without continued interventions, the likelihood of proper self-management is reduced. **Table 3** outlines important points that should be covered with the patient on each visit.

Opportunities for Collaborative Practice in the Management of Asthma

As a pharmacist, you can play a role in the management of asthma by supporting patients, identifying their unique needs, and providing ongoing education. Asthma is often undertreated and may be undiagnosed. Common reasons for the underdiagnosis and undertreatment of asthma are listed in **Table 4**.[7] A pharmacist who recognizes that a patient is using over-the-counter respiratory inhalers or other agents can triage the patient and refer him or her to a physician or other health care provider for further workup of symptoms.

Many patients today seek more than one individual to help them with their health-related problems. Pharmacists may serve as the coordinator of a patient's health care team. In addition, patients may be using alternative medicines or treatments in the management of their disease. It will be important to gather this information from a patient and incorporate the information in the overall treatment plan as well as communicate the information to other members of the health care team. Patients who have signs and symptoms of poorly controlled disease should be educated and referred to their health care provider for modification of therapy or additional evaluation.

Table 3. Important Patient Evaluation Points

Discuss concerns the patient might have

Review medication administration technique

Review peak flow monitoring

Review use of each medication and expected outcome

Review asthma management action plan and modify as necessary

Clarify questions

Determine level of family/peer social support

Table 4. Causes of Underdiagnosis and Undertreatment of Asthma[7]

Asthma not recognized

Low expectation from therapy

Benefits and risks of therapy poorly understood

Chronic nature of disease not appreciated

Severity of episode not recognized

Signs of worsening symptoms not recognized

Episodes treated suboptimally

Triggers not recognized

Triggers not avoided

Establishing a Professional Relationship

In the *Ambulatory Care Clinical Skills Program: Core Module*, you read several suggestions for developing a collaborative patient-pharmacist relationship. The principles discussed in the *Core Module* are applicable in pediatric and adult asthma patients alike. These strategies include acknowledging the patient promptly, maintaining eye contact with the patient, providing an overview of your role and expertise with asthma, and working to establish a trusting relationship. When possible, discussion should take place in a quiet and private area to maintain patient confidentiality. Establishing your role with the patient as a partner in his or her ongoing care will be helpful in building a trusting relationship. The patient needs to be assured that you are interested in his or her overall well-being and will work with him or her to best manage the disease. Patients will want to hear that you have developed an expertise in the management of asthma. Always remember to ask patients about concerns they have regarding the disease or treatment. **Table 5** presents questions you may want to incorporate into your interview as you assess a patient.[8]

For pediatric patients, it will be important to acknowledge their uniqueness among their peers. Peer pressure can be especially difficult to deal with and should not be discounted. Asthma patients typically have to take chronic medications to prevent and control symptoms and may have to avoid social situations (such as smoking) that could trigger an asthma exacerbation. Taking chronic medications and needing to avoid situations where there is secondhand smoke can make a child feel awkward and certainly different from his or her peers. What can you do as a pharmacist to help in this situation?

First, it is OK to admit that having asthma is not fun. It is important to encourage pediatric patients to recognize that with proper management, asthma shouldn't interfere with most normal activities. You need to make certain that pediatric patients understand the potential seriousness of asthma and recognize that nonadherence to prescribed regimens or exposure to triggers may place them in a life-threatening position. This point will need to be continually reinforced with each visit because pediatric patients, especially adolescents, often feel invincible and cannot fully grasp the concept of their own mortality. Parents of young pediatric patients and adolescent patients need to be encouraged to tell the patient's friends, family, teachers, and coaches that the child has asthma and may need to use an inhaler. Making sure others are aware of the potential for an asthma exacerbation may help the pediatric patient feel less embarrassed or less awkward when the sudden need to use medication arises. Parents need to be closely involved in the management of younger patients and will need to be supportive of the older pediatric patient's treatment plan. It will be necessary to form an alliance between the patient, health care provider, and parent/caregiver.

Table 5. Assessment Questions[8]

Do you agree with the diagnosis of asthma?

How serious do you feel your asthma is?

How important is your health to you?

Do you think your asthma treatment plan and medications will work?

Are you concerned about medication side effects?

Do you think you will be able to carry out the asthma treatment plan?

Strategies for forming a relationship with an adult patient with asthma will be no different than those described in the *Core Module*. Again, patients' perceptions of their own health, seriousness of the disease, and mortality will strongly influence their behavior and adherence to a suggested treatment plan. Determining the patient's desires and quality of life goals and incorporating them into the treatment plan will help gain acceptance. If an adult caregiver is involved with a patient, it will be necessary to make sure that this person is aware of the treatment plan and triggers and is comfortable with all aspects of care that the patient may need.

Case Study

Let's consider the case of Jeremy Morgan. A woman approaches the counter.

MRS. MORGAN:
"Hello. My friend Amy suggested I talk with a pharmacist about Jeremy's asthma. She said you helped her with her own asthma. Jeremy has had asthma since he was about 2 or 3 years old, but it seems to have gotten much worse lately and I'm scared."

PHARMACIST:
"Well, I'd certainly like to try and help you with the management of Jeremy's asthma. Adolescence can be a difficult time for children with asthma. My name is Jennifer Loudon and I am a pharmacist with a lot of experience taking care of patients with asthma, especially pediatric patients. Why don't we go and sit down in the conference room where it is quiet and we can talk in private."

Mrs. Morgan and the pharmacist go into the conference room to discuss Mrs. Morgan's concerns.

PHARMACIST:
"I'd like to start filling out a record on Jeremy while we are talking. What is your full name? And Jeremy's date of birth and current weight?"

MRS. MORGAN:
"I'm sorry, my name would be helpful. It's Sally Morgan. Jeremy was born on January 13, 1986. He weighs 95 pounds. I am so scared that he is going to get really sick I don't know what to do."

PHARMACIST:
"I think that we should be able to make sense of what's going on with Jeremy. Asthma can be a scary disease, especially when it's not well controlled. I understand your concerns about Jeremy. When asthma is controlled, it shouldn't keep anyone from living a normal life. Jeremy may just be adjusting as he gets older and is no longer a child. Who is Jeremy's physician? When was Jeremy first diagnosed with asthma?"

MRS. MORGAN:
"Jeremy's doctor is Dr. Lefton. She has been his pediatrician since he was born and has always treated his asthma. Jeremy hadn't had an asthma exacerbation for several years. In the last 9 months he has experienced several exacerbations. He uses Azmacort every day and has a Proventil inhaler for emergency use. He just doesn't seem to listen to me anymore when I remind him to take his medications."

PHARMACIST:
"Being a teenager can be difficult enough these days without having a chronic disease on top of it. Kids just don't want to be singled out or seen as different. Many times kids Jeremy's age will stop taking their medications when they are around their friends because they are embarrassed and don't want to look sickly. We need to encourage Jeremy to take control of his disease and be responsible for his medications. We also need to make sure he understands the implications of an asthma exacerbation. The fact that asthma can be deadly when not treated properly is a difficult concept for anyone, especially a teenager. I'd like to set up a time to talk with Jeremy about his medications and how they should be used. I'll also review with him things that can trigger an exacerbation. I can work with him and see how he feels about his asthma and what he wants from his medications. At this age, it would be good to have Jeremy speak with me alone at first. This can give him some space and allow him to start to feel responsible for taking care of his asthma. At the end of our session, I'd like for you to come in and we can all talk a little further."

MRS. MORGAN:
"I would really appreciate having you talk with him. It would be great to have him here without me. You know how it is with young boys; all of a sudden they are embarrassed to

be seen with their mothers. I don't want him to feel like a baby. How long do you think your meeting will take? I can leave work early, drop him off, and then come in at the end like you suggested."

PHARMACIST:
"Let's plan on 20–30 minutes for our first visit. How about next Wednesday at 3:30 p.m.?"

As you read through this case, you can identify the elements of the encounter that allowed the pharmacist to begin establishing a relationship with Mrs. Morgan. The pharmacist was friendly, and she indicated what her role would be and that she had had experience with pediatric patients. The majority of communication took place in a private area, and the pharmacist indicated an interest in Jeremy by asking questions and beginning to formulate a patient record. She also acknowledged that the management of asthma becomes difficult in older children. Mrs. Morgan seemed to understand that having Jeremy meet with the pharmacist alone would be helpful. When the pharmacist meets with Jeremy, she will need to gain his trust by not demanding that he adhere to his asthma regimen. She will need to ask Jeremy how he feels about his asthma and what, if anything, he would change. She should also encourage Jeremy to avoid things that can trigger an exacerbation and help him think of strategies to make living with asthma more tolerable. Jeremy will be more likely to agree with a treatment plan if he feels like he is part of the decision-making process and that everyone is keeping his interests, including his social life, in mind.

Practice Example

Read the following example and think about how you would handle this patient and begin a professional relationship.

You are a pharmacist working in a retail setting, and you notice a customer who is breathing quite heavily and looking at the nonprescription inhalers. As the pharmacist, you decide to approach the patient and offer to help.

PHARMACIST JONES:
"Hello, I'm Bob Jones, the pharmacist. Is there anything that I can help you with? I see you are looking at inhalers. Is this for you or someone else?"

Mr. Kelley looks up in surprise and begins to shake his head.

MR. KELLEY:
"I sure would like to have you help me. I am so confused about what to take. I had asthma as a kid, but I outgrew that. But lately I've had trouble breathing during the day when I'm at work. I thought maybe one of these inhaler things might just do the trick. Which one do you think works the best?"

How would you respond to Mr. Kelley? What would you do to establish a professional relationship with this patient?

Obviously, the pharmacist will need to gather more information to try and understand why Mr. Kelley is having difficulty breathing. The pharmacist may need to have Mr. Kelley see his doctor rather than recommending any treatment. The pharmacist will need to find out from Mr. Kelley how long he has had symptoms and if they get better when he leaves work. The pharmacist may want to see Mr. Kelley for a formal asthma counseling session if his doctor decides he is having difficulty with asthma again.

One possible scenario may go as follows.

PHARMACIST:
"We may want to talk a little about what is causing your breathing problems before I recommend anything. Would you like to come back to the pharmacy where we will be able to talk a bit more privately?"

Mr. Kelley and the pharmacist move back to the pharmacy.

PHARMACIST:
"How long have you been having difficulty with breathing at work?"

MR. KELLEY:
"Well, I guess about a month or more. It all began in early April when my shop moved into a new building because we added a new line of products and needed to expand. I'm OK for the first hour or so, but by lunchtime I am ready to go outside for fresh air. Then I seem to do OK until it's quitting time. I just cough a lot. I just get a little nervous because my chest feels tight. I know it can't be asthma because my mother said I outgrew it."

PHARMACIST:
"It certainly sounds as though something at work may be causing you to have problems breathing.

Do you work around a lot of chemicals or fumes? Sometimes these things can irritate your airways and cause you to have symptoms of asthma. Do you ever have problems breathing when you are not at work?"

Mr. Kelley:
"Oh, I work in a chemical processing plant. I'm in charge of time study. Once in a while, I have a little trouble breathing at home, but it isn't anything like when I'm at work."

Pharmacist:
"I think your family doctor may want to know about the problems you are having breathing at work. I think that may be the best thing rather than buying one of these inhalers. It would probably be a good idea to call your doctor today and let him or her know everything you just told me. Something at work may very well be causing your asthma to act up. Most people really don't outgrow asthma; some people just don't have as many problems as they get older. It would also be a good idea to let your doctor know to make sure there is nothing else causing your breathing problems. Do you think you will be able to get in touch with your doctor today?"

Mr. Kelley:
"Oh sure, I'm off the rest of today and the next 2 days. I'll call when I get home. I appreciate your time. I guess I just needed someone to tell me I should have this checked out. I thought asthma was just a kid's problem!"

Pharmacist:
"I'll tell you what; I'd like to know what happens after you see the doctor. If need be, we can sit down and talk about what he's told you. If you have any trouble breathing between now and when you see your doctor, call the doctor right away or go to the emergency room."

This encounter illustrates how the pharmacist collected some information and used it to triage the patient to his health care provider. The pharmacist encouraged the patient to talk about his symptoms and then validated his concerns.

Summary

Asthma can be a serious, chronic disease if not properly managed and controlled. The incidence of asthma continues to grow in the United States.

Asthma affects people of all ages, from the very young to the very old. The economic and societal impact of uncontrolled asthma is tremendous. Pharmacists have an excellent opportunity to become involved with the management of these patients by offering support, education, and encouragement for appropriately managing the disease. Pharmacists need to be aware of the appropriate techniques for establishing rapport and trust with patients.

References

1. Centers for Disease Control. Fastats. Available at: www.cdc.gov/nchswww/fastats/asthma.htm. Accessed January 4, 1999.
2. American Lung Association (Epidemiology and Statistics Unit). Trends in asthma morbidity and mortality. American Lung Association Website November 1998.
3. National Heart, Lung, and Blood Institute. Expert Panel Report 2: Guidelines for the diagnosis and management of asthma. July 1997.
4. Rich M, Schneider L. Managing asthma with the adolescent. *Curr Opin Pediatr* 1996;8:301–9.
5. Bender B MH, Rand C. Nonadherence in asthmatic patients: is there a solution to the problem? *Ann Allergy Asthma Immunol* 1997;79:177–86.
6. Kelly HW, Kamada AK. Asthma. In: DiPiro JT, Talbert RL, Yee GC, et al., editors. *Pharmacotherapy: A Pathophysiologic Approach*. Stamford, CT: Appleton & Lange; 1997. p. 553–90.
7. National Asthma Education and Prevention Program. Role of the pharmacist in improving asthma care. *Am J Health-Syst Pharm* 1995;52:1411–6.
8. Geppert EF, Collazo S. Establishing a partnership with the patient with asthma. *J Allergy Clin Immunol* 1998;101:S405–8.

Self-Study Questions

Objective

Explain disease influences on pharmacist-patient relationships.

1. Describe the epidemiology of asthma.

2. List factors that may contribute to fluctuation of asthma symptoms.

3. Explain differences in asthma in adults and children.

Objective

Explain the emotional or physical characteristics of ambulatory care patients with asthma that may affect the establishment of a collaborative patient-pharmacist relationship.

4. Explain emotional characteristics of ambulatory care patients with asthma that may affect the establishment of a collaborative patient-pharmacist relationship.

5. Explain physical characteristics of ambulatory care patients with asthma that may affect the establishment of a collaborative patient-pharmacist relationship.

6. Explain how a patient's inability to understand the potential seriousness of asthma affects the establishment of a collaborative patient-pharmacist relationship.

Objective

When given a description of an ambulatory care patient with asthma, design an effective strategy for establishing a collaborative professional relationship with that patient.

Use the following case for question 7:

Joe Arnold is a 65-year-old man who has just moved to the retirement community down the road. He comes into your pharmacy and throws an albuterol inhaler on the counter. He just went to the doctor and said the doctor gave him this breathing thing. He tells you the doctor told him he had something like asthma. He thinks the doctor must be crazy. He's always been healthy as a horse. Only a little bit of trouble breathing this past fall. He tells you he's had a lot of colds lately, but he does not feel he has asthma.

7. Describe the design of an effective strategy for establishing a collaborative professional relationship with Mr. Arnold.

Use the following case for question 8:

Sally Wheeler and her mother come into your ambulatory asthma clinic. Sally is an 11-year-old girl with a recent diagnosis of asthma. She appears quite sullen and refuses to look at you. Her mother appears frustrated and asks you to help them with Sally's asthma.

8. Describe the design of an effective strategy for establishing a collaborative professional relationship with Sally Wheeler and her mother.

Use the following case for question 9:

Mr. Mitchell comes into your pharmacy clinic with his 6-year-old son, Collin. He and his wife were recently divorced; he shares custody of Collin with his wife. Collin was rushed to the emergency room earlier in the week after having difficulty breathing during a little league football game. Mr. Mitchell thinks he remembers Collin having breathing difficulty in the past. The doctor told Mr. Mitchell that Collin has asthma. Mr. Mitchell is obviously quite nervous. He is really concerned that his wife will blame him for letting Collin catch asthma. Collin is shy and appears withdrawn.

9. Describe the design of an effective strategy for establishing a collaborative professional relationship with Collin and his family.

Self-Study Answers

1. Asthma, a chronic respiratory condition, affects approximately 14.6 million Americans. Approximately one third of patients with asthma are children <18 years of age. The prevalence of asthma has continued to rise significantly in all age groups, including children. An estimated 5500 deaths each year in the United States are attributed to asthma. Asthma-related mortality occurs more frequently among African Americans than among white Americans.

2. The severity of a patient's asthma may fluctuate. This fluctuation reflects varying control of inflammatory episodes and may be attributed to seasonal triggers, environmental factors, understanding of the disease, exercise, infections, compliance with medications, and other health conditions.

3. Childhood asthma is most often associated with atopy, viral illness, or allergies. Adult-onset asthma does not have a clear association with allergy. Some adult patients have allergies, other patients in this age group have asthma that is associated with nasal polyps and aspirin sensitivity, work-related exposures, or chronic sinusitis.

4. Patients with asthma may have a number of emotional characteristics that could affect the development of a collaborative professional relationship. These characteristics include a desire to not stand out or be different from others, failure to recognize severity of the disease, down-playing potential consequences of poorly controlled disease, and rebellion during the adolescent years.

5. Patients with asthma do not look any different from other patients. Physical characteristics that may affect the development of a collaborative professional relationship include conditions that impair medication administration or monitoring. Two examples would be a young patient who has difficulty coordinating medication administration and monitoring devices and patients with arthritis, who may have the same difficulty.

6. It will be difficult to gain acceptance of a treatment plan and commitment to adhere to a prescribed treatment plan in patients that fail to comprehend the potential for serious morbidity and mortality associated with poorly controlled asthma. The episodic nature of asthma, with periods of few or no symptoms, may lull patients into believing that asthma is nothing to be concerned about.

7. It will be necessary to gain Mr. Arnold's trust and acknowledge that it must be frustrating to be told that you may have an illness when you have always been healthy. Acknowledging that Mr. Arnold has moved to a new community and recently retired and thus has had many changes in his life will also be important. It will be important to let Mr. Arnold know about your expertise in the area of asthma education. You will want to inform him about the incidence of asthma in his age group and let him know that some patients do not develop signs and symptoms of asthma until they are older. You will need to find out from Mr. Arnold what his concerns about asthma are and help him understand that if he takes appropriate precautions, having asthma should not interfere with his life.

8. You will want to talk with Mrs. Wheeler and Sally about your expertise in the area of asthma. Offering to take them to a more private area to talk will be necessary, especially because Sally does not appear to appreciate being towed around by her mother. Because Sally is a preteen, you may want to offer talking with her alone first. Part of the problem may be that Sally is going through so many changes in her life at the moment that she is feeling awkward and would benefit from a one-on-one conversation with you. Sally could be concerned about being different from the rest of her friends and classmates. You will need to work with her and help her understand the importance of controlling her asthma. You will need to reassure Sally that asthma that is well controlled shouldn't set her apart from anyone in her class. She will be able to participate in all of the same activities. Teaching her about her medications and helping her decide on a schedule that best meets her health needs and is least intrusive in her life will be necessary.

9. In this case, you will need to explain your expertise in the area of pediatric asthma and acknowledge the difficult circumstances that

Mr. Mitchell finds himself in. You should offer to provide him with basic asthma education both for himself and his ex-wife. You will need to let him know that it will be especially important for Collin's health that he and his ex-wife both understand the basics about asthma and how to best help Collin. Mr. Mitchell may be concerned that Collin won't be able to play sports, but you will need to let him know that with adequately controlled asthma Collin's physical activities should not be limited.

Creating a Patient-Specific Database
Part 1: Specific Physical Assessment Skills

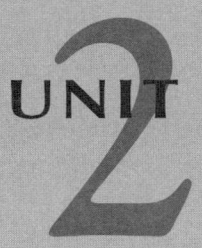
UNIT 2

Unit Objectives	18
Unit Organization	18
Physical Assessment Procedures Used in the Evaluation of Ambulatory Care Patients with Asthma	18
Assessing General Appearance	18
Vital Signs	19
Expanded Respiratory Evaluation	22
Pulmonary Function Testing	25
Peak Flow Monitoring	26
Case Study	29
Practice Example	30
Summary	30
References	31
Self-Study Questions	32
Self-Study Answers	33

Asthma is a variable disease. Although there are some identifiable unifying characteristics, each individual's asthma course is unique and episodic. This variability in symptoms and presentation makes the evaluation of a patient with asthma complex. No single physical finding or reported symptom will define the next steps of action; rather, a comprehensive medical and symptom history must be combined with physical assessment of the patient. Pharmacists often obtain the results of these examinations from the records of other health care practitioners. The expanded role of pharmacists in the management of asthma patients necessitates that pharmacists have a thorough knowledge of how to perform a physical examination of a patient with asthma.

The Ambulatory Care Clinical Skills Program: Core Module provided you with the knowledge necessary to assess a patient's vital signs and general appearance. In this unit, you will learn how to assess respiratory status in more detail than was presented in the *Core Module*, using a stethoscope to listen for respiratory sounds. This unit will also introduce pulmonary function testing.

Competence in assessment of vital signs and general appearance is gained by repetitive hands-on demonstration and practice with trained educators.

Unit Objectives

After you successfully complete this unit, you will be able to:
- state physical assessment procedures that are routinely conducted for ambulatory care patients with asthma;
- explain the role of the various types of physical assessment information required for the database of ambulatory care patients with asthma in planning their pharmaceutical care;
- explain factors unique to ambulatory care patients with asthma when interpreting their general appearance;
- explain correct technique for using a stethoscope to examine an ambulatory care asthma patient;
- explain correct technique for the use of a peak flow meter; and
- when given the results of a physical assessment of an ambulatory care patient with asthma, accurately interpret the results.

Unit Organization

This unit will begin with an overview of pertinent physical findings that aid in the assessment of the patient with asthma. We will then focus on expanded respiratory evaluation, discussing correct use of the stethoscope to listen for breath sounds. We will discuss pulmonary function testing, including correct use of a peak flow meter in examining the patient with asthma. Last, you will learn how to accurately interpret results from the physical assessment of an ambulatory care patient with asthma.

Physical Assessment Procedures Used in the Evaluation of Ambulatory Care Patients with Asthma

The presentation of a patient with asthma will depend on both the severity of the underlying disease and the presence of an acute exacerbation of the disease. Each time a patient with asthma is seen, a detailed history should be gathered from the patient and a cursory review of the general appearance of the patient must be done. Specific physical assessment techniques will be used, depending on the evaluation of those findings and the purpose of the visit. Although the subject is not covered in this unit, keep in mind how the patient's current pharmacologic treatments may correlate with physical findings. For example, a patient may be jittery and shaky after using a $beta_2$-adrenergic agonist inhaler.

The patient with asthma should be interviewed and examined in a calm and private environment, as described in the *Core Module*. The physical environment is particularly important in the evaluation of a patient with asthma because the respiratory distress associated with exacerbations of the disease frequently makes the patient anxious. Children should be examined with their parents present; as often as possible, small children should be seated on their parents' laps during the exam.

Assessing General Appearance

Physical examination of a patient with asthma begins with an assessment of general appearance.

The *Core Module* provides a good overview of this observational technique. **Figure 1** lists some specific findings that signal the need for a more extensive evaluation of a patient. A patient who is disoriented or confused may not be providing adequate oxygen to the brain as a result of extreme respiratory distress. An asthma patient experiencing an acute exacerbation will have difficulty breathing. Patients in respiratory distress will use short phrases or single words to conserve their energy. They will prefer sitting to lying because this position makes it easier for them to use accessory muscles for breathing. The patient may exhibit diaphoresis in response to difficulty breathing. Bluish color of the skin or in the nail beds is associated with hypoxia, although the absence of this finding does not eliminate the possibility of hypoxia. Patients whose asthma is severe may exhibit signs of chronic hypoventilation: clubbing or dullness and flatness of the fingertips.

Asthma is frequently associated with upper respiratory infections. Patients should be questioned about symptoms such as runny nose and congestion. Sinusitis is also common among patients with asthma. Signs and symptoms of sinusitis are outlined in **Table 1**.[1] Another nasal finding common among patients with asthma is nasal polyps.

The association of asthma with allergy is also common. Some patients with asthma will have manifestations of increased dermatological sensitivity, such as eczema, in addition to respiratory symptoms. **Figure 2** provides a sheet to record general appearance findings.

Vital Signs

It will be important to have a record of a patient's weight and height. These assessments are particularly important in the asthma patient population because a significant proportion of your patients will be children. Weight will be important for dosing some medications in both the pediatric and the adult population. Height and weight will be important measures to follow to assess whether the pediatric patient is growing appropriately. An assessment of respiratory rate, pulse, and blood pressure will be warranted at some visits. Specific instances that may require an assessment of vital signs include patient complaints of not feeling right, a general assessment of the patient that indicates potential respiratory distress, or a planned physical examination that has been scheduled. It is important to recognize that between acute exacerbations of the disease, the physical examination of a patient with asthma does not reveal significant physical findings. Often, it is the patient or parent interview that provides more insight into the patient's clinical status. During a routine visit, patients in no apparent distress will need a baseline recording of these vital signs as a comparison for future visits.

Respiratory rates increase in patients experiencing an exacerbation of their asthma, and their breaths are shallow. The presence of a slow respiratory rate in a person with asthma is an ominous finding. This slow rate can signal exhaustion and impending respiratory failure when corroborated with other findings. Normal respiratory rate varies by the patient's size and age, as outlined in the *Core Module*. **Table 2** contains normal respiratory rates for adult and pediatric patients.[2]

Pulse rate also varies by the patient's age; normal values for pediatric patients are listed in **Table 3**.[3] The technique for obtaining a pulse is

Table 1. Signs and Symptoms of Sinusitis[1]

Tenderness over sinus cavities (worsens with movement)

Headache (pressure in head) that does not respond well to analgesics

Runny nose (discharge frequently purulent)

Fever

Abnormal decrease in sensitivity to odors

Table 2. Normal Respiratory Rate by Age[2]

Age	Rate (Breaths/Minute)
Newborn	30–60
Infant (1–6 months)	30–40
Infant (6–12 months)	24–30
1–4 years	20–30
4–6 years	20–25
6–12 years	16–20
12 years and older	12–16

Assessment of General Appearance

Patient _____ Date _____

General Appearance	Observations and Comments

Level of consciousness
    alertness: alert, confused, delirious, stuporous, comatose,
    orientation: person, place, time
	Confusion, disorientation

Signs of distress respiratory distress, pain, anxiety, etc.	Respiratory distress
Posture, motor activity, and gait Describe	Reluctant to lie flat; prefers sitting, hunched shoulders
Dress, grooming, and personal hygiene Describe	

Affect
    normal, inappropriate
    Describe
	Nervousness, anxiety

Speech
    normal, impaired
    Describe
	Uses shortened phrases or single words

Skin
    color: normal, blue, brown, red, pallor
    texture: normal, coarse, dry, oily
    turgor: good, poor
    edema
    lesions: color, type, configuration, anatomic distribution, consistency
	Bluish color to skin, nail beds, perioral area, sweating

Shown are specific findings that signal the need for a more extensive evaluation of an asthma patient.

Figure 1. General appearance and vital signs

Assessment of General Appearance

Patient _____ Date _____

General Appearance	Observations and Comments

Level of consciousness
    alertness: alert, confused, delirious, stuporous, comatose,
    orientation: person, place, time	

Signs of distress respiratory distress, pain, anxiety, etc.	
Posture, motor activity, and gait *Describe*	
Dress, grooming, and personal hygiene *Describe*	

Affect
    normal, inappropriate
    Describe	

Speech
    normal, impaired
    Describe	

Skin
    color: normal, blue, brown, red, pallor
    texture: normal, coarse, dry, oily
    turgor: good, poor
    edema
    lesions: color, type, configuration, anatomic distribution, consistency	

Figure 2. General appearance and vital signs

Table 3. Normal Pediatric Pulse Rate by Age[3]

Age	Mean Heart Rate (Beats/Minute)	Heart Rate Range (2nd—98th Percentile)
<1 d	123	93–154
1–2 d	123	91–159
3–6 d	129	91–166
1–3 wk	148	107–182
1–2 mo	149	121–179
3–5 mo	141	106–186
6–11 mo	134	109–169
1–2 y	119	89–151
3–4 y	108	73–137
5–7 y	100	65–133
8–11 y	91	62–130
12–15 y	85	60–119

outlined in the *Core Module*. In an infant, a brachial pulse may be used in place of the radial pulse because it is easier to palpate. Patients experiencing an acute exacerbation of their asthma are frequently tachycardic. Tachycardia is present as a result of the actions of catecholamines released in response to impaired gas exchange.

Unit 4 of the *Core Module* provides an excellent review of blood pressure measurement, which in the young pediatric patient requires expertise. Accurate measurement requires specialized blood pressure cuffs. Even with an appropriately sized cuff, it may be difficult to obtain a blood pressure measurement from an uncooperative child. Normal pediatric blood pressures are listed in **Table 4**.[4] Blood pressure may be elevated in the patient with asthma in acute distress as a result of increased catecholamine concentrations. The older pediatric patient or adult in distress may exhibit pulsus paradoxus, the drop in systolic blood pressure that occurs with inspiration. Pulsus paradoxus has been correlated with worsening condition; a drop in blood pressure of 10–20 mmHg represents moderate distress, and a drop of >20 mmHg represents significant respiratory distress.[2] The absence of this finding does not rule out asthma or an exacerbation of asthma.

Expanded Respiratory Evaluation

Your current practice site will determine whether you will be able to do an expanded respiratory evaluation. You will need to be able to examine patients who have been stripped of clothing to their waist. The patient should be seated for this examination. You will first examine the patient in the seated position to observe the patient for evidence of accessory muscle use in breathing. Posture should be noted; hunched shoulders may be a sign of respiratory difficulty. Patients experiencing respiratory difficulty frequently enlist surrounding musculature to aid in breathing. This effort includes the intercostal, suprasternal, and supraclavicular muscles. The use of accessory muscles is necessary because the chest cavity is hyperexpanded and the diaphragm is lowered. Hyperexpansion of the thorax is especially common among children.

Auscultation of breath sounds requires an understanding of how and where to place a stethoscope on the chest, and knowledge of normal breath sounds. The patient's positioning and cooperation are necessary to ensure accurate evaluation of breath sounds. Observe the following when performing auscultation[5]:

- To listen across the back, the patient should lean forward with arms folded.

Table 4. Normal Pediatric Blood Pressure Curves

Age (years)	Blood Pressure Percentile[a]	Systolic BP (mmHg) by Percentile of Height[b]							Diastolic BP (mmHg) by Percentile of Height[b]						
		5%	10%	25%	50%	75%	90%	95%	5%	10%	25%	50%	75%	90%	95%
Boys															
1	90th	94	95	97	98	100	102	102	50	51	52	53	54	54	55
	95th	98	99	101	102	104	106	106	55	55	56	57	58	59	59
2	90th	98	99	100	102	104	105	106	55	55	56	57	58	59	59
	95th	101	102	104	106	108	109	110	59	59	60	61	62	63	63
3	90th	100	101	103	105	107	108	109	59	59	60	61	62	63	63
	95th	104	105	107	109	111	112	113	63	63	64	65	66	67	67
4	90th	102	103	105	107	109	110	111	62	62	63	64	65	66	66
	95th	106	107	109	111	113	114	115	66	67	67	68	69	70	71
5	90th	104	105	106	108	110	112	112	65	65	66	67	68	69	69
	95th	108	109	110	112	114	115	116	69	70	70	71	72	73	74
6	90th	105	106	108	110	111	113	114	67	68	69	70	70	71	72
	95th	109	110	112	114	115	117	117	72	72	73	74	75	76	76
7	90th	106	107	109	111	113	114	115	69	70	71	72	72	73	74
	95th	110	111	113	115	116	118	119	74	74	75	76	77	78	78
8	90th	107	108	110	112	114	115	116	71	71	72	73	74	75	75
	95th	111	112	114	116	118	119	120	75	76	76	77	78	79	80
9	90th	109	110	112	113	115	117	117	72	73	73	74	75	76	77
	95th	113	114	116	117	119	121	121	76	77	78	79	80	80	81
10	90th	110	112	113	115	117	118	119	73	74	74	75	76	77	78
	95th	114	115	117	119	121	122	123	77	78	79	80	80	81	82
11	90th	112	113	115	117	119	120	121	74	74	75	76	77	78	78
	95th	116	117	119	121	123	124	125	78	79	79	80	81	82	83
12	90th	115	116	117	119	121	123	123	75	75	76	77	78	78	79
	95th	119	120	121	123	125	126	127	79	79	80	81	82	83	83
13	90th	117	118	120	122	124	125	126	75	76	76	77	78	79	80
	95th	121	122	124	126	128	129	130	79	80	81	82	83	83	84
14	90th	120	121	123	125	126	128	128	76	76	77	78	79	80	80
	95th	124	125	127	128	130	132	132	80	81	81	82	83	84	85
15	90th	123	124	125	127	129	131	131	77	77	78	79	80	81	81
	95th	127	128	129	131	133	134	135	81	82	83	83	84	85	86
16	90th	125	126	128	130	132	133	134	79	79	80	81	82	82	83
	95th	129	130	132	134	136	137	138	83	83	84	85	86	87	87
17	90th	128	129	131	133	134	136	136	81	81	82	83	84	85	85
	95th	132	133	135	136	138	140	140	85	85	86	87	88	89	89
Girls															
1	90th	97	98	99	100	102	103	104	53	53	53	54	55	56	56
	95th	101	102	103	104	105	107	107	57	57	57	58	59	60	60
2	90th	99	99	100	102	103	104	105	57	57	58	58	59	60	61
	95th	102	103	104	105	107	108	109	61	61	62	62	63	64	65
3	90th	100	100	102	103	104	105	106	61	61	61	62	63	63	64
	95th	104	104	105	107	108	109	110	65	65	65	66	67	67	68

continued on next page

Table 4. Normal Pediatric Blood Pressure Curves (cont.)

Age (years)	Blood Pressure Percentile[a]	Systolic BP (mmHg) by Percentile of Height[b]							Diastolic BP (mmHg) by Percentile of Height[b]						
		5%	10%	25%	50%	75%	90%	95%	5%	10%	25%	50%	75%	90%	95%

Girls (cont.)

Age	Percentile	5%	10%	25%	50%	75%	90%	95%	5%	10%	25%	50%	75%	90%	95%
4	90th	101	102	103	104	106	107	108	63	63	64	65	65	66	67
	95th	105	106	107	108	109	111	111	67	67	68	69	69	70	71
5	90th	103	103	104	106	107	108	109	65	66	66	67	68	68	69
	95th	107	107	108	110	111	112	113	69	70	70	71	72	72	73
6	90th	104	105	106	107	109	110	111	67	67	68	69	69	70	71
	95th	108	109	110	111	112	114	114	71	71	72	73	73	74	75
7	90th	106	107	108	109	110	112	112	69	69	69	70	71	72	72
	95th	110	110	112	113	114	115	116	73	73	73	74	75	76	76
8	90th	108	109	110	111	112	113	114	70	70	71	71	72	73	74
	95th	112	112	113	115	116	117	118	74	74	75	75	76	77	78
9	90th	110	110	112	113	114	115	116	71	72	72	73	74	74	75
	95th	114	114	115	117	118	119	120	75	76	76	77	78	78	79
10	90th	112	112	114	115	116	117	118	73	73	73	74	75	76	76
	95th	116	116	117	119	120	121	122	77	77	77	78	79	80	80
11	90th	114	114	116	117	118	119	120	74	74	75	75	76	77	77
	95th	118	118	119	121	122	123	124	78	78	79	79	80	81	81
12	90th	116	116	118	119	120	121	122	75	75	76	76	77	78	78
	95th	120	120	121	123	124	125	126	79	79	80	80	81	82	82
13	90th	118	118	119	121	122	123	124	76	76	77	78	78	79	80
	95th	121	122	123	125	126	127	128	80	80	81	82	82	83	84
14	90th	119	120	121	122	124	125	126	77	77	78	79	79	80	81
	95th	123	124	125	126	128	129	130	81	81	82	83	83	84	85
15	90th	121	121	122	124	125	126	127	78	78	79	79	80	81	82
	95th	124	125	126	128	129	130	131	82	82	83	83	84	85	86
16	90th	122	122	123	125	126	127	128	79	79	79	80	81	82	82
	95th	125	126	127	128	130	131	132	83	83	83	84	85	86	86
17	90th	122	123	124	125	126	128	128	79	79	79	80	81	82	82
	95th	126	126	127	129	130	131	132	83	83	83	84	85	86	86

[a]Blood pressure percentile determined by a single measurement.
[b]Height percentile determined by standard growth curves.

Source: reprinted with permission from reference 4.

- To listen at the anterior chest, the patient should sit erect.
- The patient should take slow, deep breaths through the mouth. You may have to demonstrate for the patient the pace and depth of these breaths.
- Place the diaphragm of the stethoscope on the chest.
- Other than the chest expansion, there should be no movement of the patient or the stethoscope while evaluating a breath.
- Listen in all quadrants of the lung fields during both inspiration and expiration.

A patient in obvious respiratory distress should not undergo this exam. Pediatric patients may need additional coaching to encourage participation. The patient can be asked to blow out an imaginary flame on your finger to encourage deep breathing. Appropriate placement of the stethoscope is illustrated in **Figure 3**.[6]

The flow of air throughout the respiratory tract produces breath sounds. Healthy lung tissue pro-

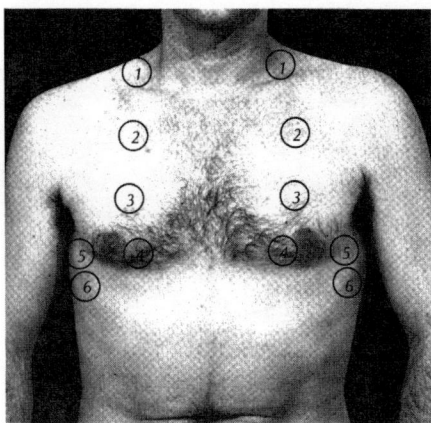

Figure 3. Appropriate placement of the stethoscope during the expanded respiratory exam.
Source: reproduced with permission from reference 6.

duces low-pitched and low-intensity sounds. The characteristic sound associated with asthma is the wheeze. Wheezing is produced by turbulent air in the obstructed airways. It is a continuous, high-pitched, almost whistle-like sound heard during inspiration and expiration. It is important to note that although the wheeze is associated classically with asthma, any condition that causes obstruction in the airways may produce wheezing. Also, it is important to remember that not every person with asthma wheezes. For many patients the only presenting symptom is cough. In addition, some patients in significant distress will not have audible wheezes because airflow is severely restricted.

Pulmonary Function Testing

Pulmonary function testing is an important component of the diagnosis of asthma. According to the National Heart, Lung, and Blood Institute Asthma Education and Prevention Program Expert Panel Report 2 released in 1997, the diagnosis of asthma requires documentation of the reversibility of airway obstruction.[7] Documentation is usually accomplished through the use of pulmonary function testing (PFT), also referred to as spirometry. PFT may also be used to track the progress of patients and their response to medications. The Expert Panel recommends PFT for asthma patients as follows:
- at initial diagnosis;
- after treatment is initiated and symptoms and peak expiratory flow have stabilized, to document attainment of near-normal airway function; and
- at least every 1–2 years to assess the maintenance of airway function.

Note that these are recommendations; not every patient with a diagnosis of asthma will have had PFT. PFT equipment will not be available in the usual ambulatory pharmacy practice site. It will be important for you in managing a patient with asthma to understand PFT results and explain them to your patients.

Asthma is an inflammatory disease that ultimately results in constriction of bronchial smooth muscle and airflow obstruction. This obstruction may be triggered by exposure to specific environmental factors. Asthma usually has some degree of diurnal variation, which is exaggerated in some patients. Patients presenting for PFT must not have been exposed to their known triggers prior to testing, nor should they have used any bronchodilating medication prior to the evaluation. Either of these situations may affect PFT results. It is also important that the time of the evaluation be noted to account for variability due to normal diurnal rhythms. In cases in which medical history is consistent with asthma and PFT results are normal or near normal, bronchoprovocation with methacholine, histamine, or exercise challenge may be attempted by specialists.[7]

Normal or predicted values for PFT are determined by defining a range of values for persons of the same age, sex, height, and race.[8] Abnormal results are defined as values outside the range that includes 95% of the variations of normal.

Patients experiencing severe symptoms or who cannot cooperate with the testing procedure do not receive PFT. Spirometry is generally useful in children over the age of 4, although some children may have difficulty with the testing until after the age of 7.[7] Testing involves the patient taking a breath that completely fills his or her lungs and then pushing the breath out as fast as possible until the lungs feel empty. This maneuver may be difficult for children, geriatric patients, and those with severe debilitation. These difficulties, in combination with costs, may exclude some asthma patients from PFT. PFT results are reported as numerical values and may also be represented graphically as a flow-volume or flow-time loop. The most commonly reported PFT values are summarized in **Table 5**.[7,8] **Figure 4** presents a graphic representation of PFT results.[7] More sophisticated PFT may be performed, and additional values may be reported. The obstructive

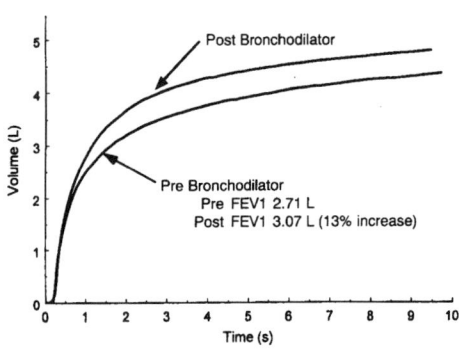
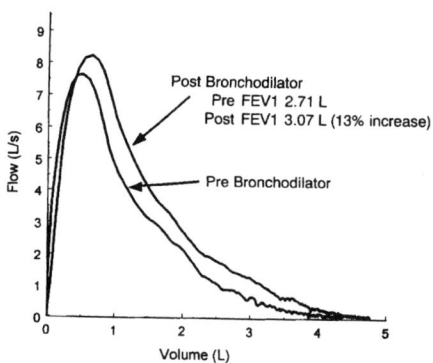

Figure 4. Peak flow testing (PFT) flow-volume results
Source: reprinted with permission from reference 7.

nature of asthmatic airways impedes the ability of the lungs to rapidly expel air. Therefore, one of the parameters studied in patients with asthma undergoing PFT is the forced expiratory volume in 1 second (FEV_1). The severity of asthma is usually defined by the percentage of the predicted FEV_1 value for persons of the same age, race, height, and sex.[8]

- FEV_1 between 60 and 75% of the predicted value is mild obstruction.
- FEV_1 between 40 and 59% of the predicted value is moderate obstruction.
- FEV_1 <40% of the predicted value is severe obstruction.

Other pulmonary diseases cause obstruction. Asthma is differentiated by the reversibility of the disease. After the first measurement of FEV_1, the patient is given an inhaled bronchodilator. Twenty minutes later, a second set of pulmonary function values is taken. An increase in FEV_1 of >12% following treatment with a bronchodilator indicates reversibility.[7]

Peak Flow Monitoring

The peak flow meter has become a frequently used device in evaluation of patients with asthma. Peak flow meters measure the largest expiratory flow that

Table 5. Pulmonary Function Test Measures[7,8]

Measure	Abbreviation	Definition
Total Lung Capacity	TLC	The volume of air in the lungs after maximal inspiration
Residual Volume	RV	The volume of air left in the lungs after maximal expiration
Vital Capacity	VC	Volume of gas exhaled during the transition from TLC to RV
Forced Vital Capacity	FVC	The volume of gas exhaled during an effort to exhale
Forced Expiratory Volume in 1 Second	FEV_1	The volume of air expired in the first second of the FVC
Forced Midexpiratory Flow	FEV_{25-75}	Average of forced expiratory flow during the middle part of the FVC
Percent FEV_1	$FEV_1\%$	$FEV_1/FVC \times 100$

is achieved with a maximally forced effort from a position of maximum inspiration.[9] Peak flow meters provide a simple, quantitative, reproducible, and objective measurement of large airway function.[10] Despite these advantages and the fact that these devices are relatively inexpensive, spirometry is generally preferred over the peak flow meter for diagnosis for several reasons[7]:

- Even the best published peak expiratory flow reference values show wide variability.
- Reference values need to be specific to each brand of peak flow meter.
- Normative brand-specific values are currently not available for most brands.

Peak flow meters are most useful when a single device is used for ongoing monitoring of an individual asthma patient. Pharmacists actively involved in the care of patients with asthma should have a good understanding of the proper use and maintenance of peak flow meters.

Many different peak flow meters are available. They come in two ranges to account for physiological differences in airway size. The low-range peak flow meter is used to examine small children. The standard peak flow meter is used for older children and adults. The American Thoracic Society has published standards for the evaluation of these devices.[11] Pharmacists involved in the management of asthma should be familiar with these standards and be able to aid patients in the selection of a device. These standards state[11]:

- A peak flow meter should be capable of generating accurate flows between 1 and 900 L/min (0–15 L/sec) and yield readings within 10% or 10 L/min of the true volume, whichever is greater.
- The repeatability (within instrument agreement) should be 3% or 10 L/min, whichever is greater.
- The reproducibility (interdevice variability) should be within 5% or 20 L/min, whichever is greater.

In addition to the traditional peak flow meter, which requires manual recording of the value achieved, electronic devices are now available that automatically record the value. Some of these devices may even be connected to a telephone line so that the stored information may be transmitted to you or another health care provider. The electronic devices are still expensive, and the slight advantage of avoiding manual recording must be weighed against this expense. Once a peak flow meter is chosen, it is important that the patient continue to use the same device for all readings.

Patients will need to understand how to use a peak flow meter. They should be encouraged to bring their flow meter with them when they come in for routine visits so that their technique can be observed. The values obtained with any flow meter are only as good as the patient's technique. Emphasize these steps when reviewing technique with patients:

1. Be sure that the sliding marker or arrow on the peak flow meter is at the bottom of the numbered scale (at zero or the lowest number on the scale).
2. Remove gum or food from the mouth.
3. Stand up straight and take as deep a breath as possible. The mouthpiece should be placed into the mouth and the lips closed tightly around the mouthpiece. Remember to keep the tongue away from the mouthpiece.
4. Blow out as hard and as quickly as possible.
5. The breath will cause the marker to move along the numbered scale. Note the number on a piece of paper.
6. Repeat steps 3–5 two more times for a total of three readings that are recorded. The numbers that are obtained should be close together.
7. Note the highest of the three recorded values.

Normal values for standard peak flow meter readings in adults are 500–700 L/min for men and 380–500 L/min for women. These normal values cover a wide range and are not the most useful measurements for monitoring patients with asthma. Patients should be encouraged to record their personal best for their chosen peak flow meter. The steps for determining personal best are outlined in **Figure 5** along with the proper technique for using a peak flow meter.[7] Once the personal best is determined, measurements that are obtained from the use of the peak flow meter are compared to the personal best and are often recorded as a percentage of personal best. These values are then incorporated into the action plan for a patient and may be used to direct interventions or modify current treatments. If the patient needs to switch to a different peak flow meter for any reason, a new personal best should be determined for the patient with the new device, because of interdevice variability.[10] Failure to do this might guide a patient to an incorrect intervention or steer him or her away from a needed intervention.

Interpretation of peak flow readings should be individualized for each patient, to aid the patient in

How To Use Your Peak Flow Meter

A peak flow meter is a device that measures how well air moves out of your lungs. During an asthma episode, the airways of the lungs usually begin to narrow slowly. The peak flow meter may tell you if there is narrowing in the airway hours—sometimes even days—before you have asthma symptoms.

By taking your medicine(s) early (before symptoms), you may be able to stop the episode quickly and avoid a severe asthma episode. Peak flow meters are used to check your asthma the way that blood pressure cuffs are used to check high blood pressure.

The peak flow meter also can be used to help you and your doctor:
- learn what makes your asthma worse,
- decide if your treatment plan is working well,
- decide when to add or stop medicine, and
- decide when to seek emergency care.

A peak flow meter is most helpful for patients who must take asthma medicine daily. Patients ages five and older are usually able to use a peak flow meter. Ask your doctor or nurse to show you how to use a peak flow meter.

How To Use Your Peak Flow Meter

Do the following five steps with your peak flow meter:

1. Move the indicator to the bottom of the numbered scale.
2. Stand up.
3. Take a deep breath, filling your lungs completely.
4. Place the mouthpiece in your mouth and close your lips around it. Do not put your tongue inside the hole.
5. Blow out as hard and as fast as you can in a single blow.

Write down the number you get. If you cough or make a mistake, don't write down the number; do the steps over again.

Repeat steps 1 through 5 two more times and write down the best of the three blows in your asthma diary.

Find Your Personal Best Peak Flow Number

Your personal best peak flow number is the highest peak flow number you can achieve over a 2- to 3-week period when your asthma is under good control. *Good control* is when you feel good and do not have any asthma symptoms.

Each patient's asthma is different, and your best peak flow may be higher or lower than the peak flow of someone of your same height, weight, and sex. This means that it is important for you to find your own personal best peak flow number. Your treatment plan needs to be based on your own personal best peak flow number.

To find your personal best peak flow number, take peak flow readings:

- at least twice a day for 2–3 weeks;
- when you wake up and between noon and 2:00 p.m.;
- before and after you take your short-acting inhaled beta$_2$-adrenergic agonist for quick relief, if you take this medicine; and
- as instructed by your doctor.

The Peak Flow Zone System

Once you know your personal best peak flow number, your doctor will give you the numbers that tell you what to do. The peak flow numbers are put into zones that are set up like a traffic light. This will help you know what to do when your peak flow number changes. Here is a description of these zones:

GREEN ZONE (more than ___ L/min [80% of your personal best number]) signals *good control*. No asthma symptoms are present. Take your medicine as usual.

YELLOW ZONE (between ___ L/min and ___ L/min [50 to <80% of your personal best number]) signals *caution*. You must take short-acting inhales beta$_2$-adrenergic agonist right away. Also, your asthma may not be under good day-to-day control. Ask your doctor if you need to change or increase your daily medicines.

RED ZONE (below ___ L/min [50% of your personal best number]) signals a *medical alert*. You must take short-acting inhales beta$_2$-adrenergic agonist (quick-relief medicine) right away. Call your doctor or emergency room and ask what to do or go directly to the hospital emergency room.

Record your personal best peak flow number and peak flow zones in your asthma diary.

Use the Diary To Keep Track of Your Peak Flow

Measure your peak flow when you wake up, *before* taking medicine. Write down your peak flow number in the diary every day, or as instructed by your doctor.

Actions To Take When Peak Flow Numbers Change

- Peak expiratory flow (PEF) goes between ___ L/min and ___ L/min (50–<80 percent of personal best, yellow zone).
  Action: Take short-acting inhaled beta$_2$-adrenergic agonist (quick-relief medicine) as prescribed by your doctor.

- PEF increases 20% or more when measured before and after taking short-acting inhaled beta$_2$-adrenergic agonist (quick-relief medicine).
  Action: Talk to your doctor about adding more medicine to control your asthma better (for example, an anti-inflammatory medication).

Figure 5. Using your peak flow meter
Source: reprinted with permission from reference 7.

self-management decisions. Knowledge of the patient's personal best will help determine how peak flow measurements are interpreted. Peak flow measurements are stratified into zones that correlate with a patient's clinical status. These zones may be color coded into a red (danger), yellow (cautionary), and green (good) zone, with a range of peak flow readings designated for each zone. The green zone is associated with peak flow readings that are 80–100% of the patient's personal best. The yellow zone is associated with peak flow readings that are 50–79% of the patient's personal best. The red zone is associated with peak flow readings of <50% of the patient's personal best.[7] The zones are used as a guideline for both patients and health care providers to monitor and identify changes in respiratory status. Based on the zone the reading falls into, a patient may be instructed to increase the dosage of a medication or add a new medication to the current regimen until peak flow readings return to the green zone.

Peak flow meter readings have a diurnal pattern. Values will be maximal around 4 p.m., and the lowest readings will occur at approximately 4 a.m. For this reason, it is important for the patient to consistently monitor peak flow readings at the same time. For some patients it will be important to document the degree of the morning dip in peak flow readings as it correlates with disease severity.[7]

Not all patients are candidates for continuous monitoring with a peak flow meter. Some patients may only require short-term monitoring of peak flow meter readings. The Expert Panel 2 Report identifies patients who will most likely benefit from peak flow meter monitoring as[7]:

- Short-term monitoring in patients with moderate to severe persistent asthma during acute exacerbations to determine the severity of the exacerbation and guide therapeutic decisions in the home, clinician's office, or emergency department.
- Long-term daily peak flow monitoring in patients with moderate to severe asthma to detect early changes in disease status, evaluate responses to changes in therapy, provide assessment of severity for patients with poor perception of airflow obstruction, and afford a quantitative measure of impairment.
- Short-term monitoring may also be useful in patients with moderate to severe asthma who do not perform long-term monitoring to evaluate changes in therapy, identify temporal relationship to potential triggers, and establish the patient's personal best.

It is important to recognize the limitations of peak flow meters and to use them appropriately. These limitations include[9]:

- the potential for unrecognized device malfunction that may lead to inappropriate therapeutic action,
- necessity for strong patient commitment to perform regular monitoring and record-keeping, and
- the potential for fungal contamination of the device if not properly maintained.

In addition, it is important to remember that a significant limitation of these devices is that they require effort and cooperation from the patient. The results recorded must be considered as one piece of information and should be assimilated with other history, physical assessment, and laboratory findings.

Case Study

Let's return to the case of Jeremy Morgan. He returns to the pharmacy for the scheduled appointment. You greet him and move with him into your office and close the door to afford some privacy. You take out the data sheet that you began following the conversation with his mother. Although the purpose of this visit is to assess educational needs, you casually observe his general appearance while initiating a conversation.

You note that he is a thin, pale boy of 13. He understands that he is here about his asthma. He appears nervous, will not make eye contact with you, and is fidgety, as though he cannot get comfortable. He gives you the Patient Database Form that he and his mother have completed. You continue to speak to him in a calm voice about school. He answers only in very short phrases or single words. He coughs occasionally.

PHARMACIST:
"Jeremy, how do you feel today?"

JEREMY:
"OK."

PHARMACIST:
"Do you feel better or worse today than yesterday?"

JEREMY:
"Same."

As you are questioning him, you can see that there is a little sweat on his upper lip.

PHARMACIST:
"Do you use a peak flow meter?"

JEREMY:
"No."

Based on Jeremy's general appearance you are anxious about his respiratory status. He has several findings that would trigger further evaluation. He is nervous and anxious, which might be simply a result of the newness of the situation or a signal of respiratory distress. His sweating could also be a result either of increased effort breathing or of nervousness. His use of simple phrases could be an effort to conserve valuable energy for breathing or simply adolescent shyness. He is stating that his overall appearance is normal for him. You are uncomfortable and ask him if it would be all right with him if you listened to him breathe. With his agreement, you continue your physical exam.

> Respiratory rate: 24 breaths per minute and shallow
> Pulse rate: 90 bpm
> Obvious use of accessory muscles; auscultation reveals audible wheezing.

The pharmacist's interpretation of these findings is that Jeremy appears to be in mild to moderate respiratory distress.

Practice Example

It's your turn to practice with Mr. Kelley. As you recall, Mr. Kelley is a 43-year-old white man who was complaining about shortness of breath at work. You sent him to his physician's office for evaluation. He returns to your pharmacy to get his prescriptions filled. He seems to want to talk with you about what happened with the physician and to get your approval of the "machine" the physician gave him to breathe into. You invite Mr. Kelley into your private office. What physical assessment data would you collect on Mr. Kelley? Write down what you would do.

Mr. Kelley's general appearance is that of a slightly overweight white male who is somewhat jittery. He has good color. He appears to be very concerned following his appointment with his physician. He asked his physician for a copy of the exam, and he gives this to you. He has no difficulty speaking. At the physician's office, the following parameters were recorded:

> Ht: 5'10"
> Wt: 186 lbs
> Respiratory rate: 20 breaths per minute
> Pulse rate: 78 bpm
> Breathing shallow
> BP: 130/80 mmHg
> Wheezing present

You note that a dose of albuterol was administered at the physician's office.

You ask if it would be OK with Mr. Kelley if you listened to his breathing yourself so that you have your own records to follow as well as the physician's.

Mr. Kelley agrees. You note the following:

> Respiratory rate: 15 and comfortable
> Pulse rate: 80
> No obvious use of accessory muscles to breathe; on auscultation, only occasional wheezing is heard.

Based on the physician's findings in his office, Mr. Kelley was probably in respiratory distress at the time of the appointment. His overall demeanor now, although he is anxious about his disease, reveals a patient breathing comfortably following bronchodilator therapy. He only occasionally wheezes. His rapid pulse may be normal or a result of the medication he's been given. Mr. Kelly appears before you at this visit having had bronchodilator therapy, and he appears to have responded positively to the medication.

Think of how important the patient history is in this case. Had you not known about Mr. Kelley's physician visit, you might have misinterpreted the results of your physical exam as a stable respiratory exam rather than a post medication exam.

Summary

Asthma is a chronic illness that is episodic in nature. It is important to have physical assessment data on the patient as well as a thorough history to make informed decisions about treatment choices. As pharmacists continue to expand their role in the outpatient management of patients with asthma, they will be more likely to record their own physical assessment data. At a minimum this will include the general appearance of the patient with asthma. Depending on the physical layout of the practice site, physical assessment may also include a more detailed evaluation of the respiratory system.

Given the results from these assessments, pharmacists will be able to appropriately educate and triage patients with asthma. Competence in assessment of vital signs and general appearance is gained by repetitive hands-on demonstration and practice with trained educators.

References

1. Richer M, LeBel M. Upper respiratory tract infections. In: DiPiro JT, Talbert RL, Yee GC, et al., editors. *Pharmacotherapy: A Pathophysiologic Approach*. Stamford, CT: Appleton & Lange; 1997. p.2017–35.
2. Gayle MO, Kissoon N. Assessment of respiratory distress in the asthmatic child: when should we be concerned? *Pediatr Ann* 1996;25:128–35.
3. Taketomo CK, Hodding JH, Kraus DM. *Pediatric Dosage Handbook*. Hudson, OH: Lexi-Comp; 1996.
4. National High Blood Pressure Education Program Working Group on Hypertension Control in Children and Adolescents. Update on the 1987 task force report on high blood pressure in children and adolescents: a working group report from the national high blood pressure education program. *Pediatrics* 1996;98:649–58.
5. Seidel HM, Ball JW, Dains JE, Benedict GW. *Mosby's Guide to Physical Examination*. St. Louis, MO: Mosby-Year Book; 1995.
6. Bates B. *A Guide To Physical Examination and History Taking* 6th ed. Philadelphia, PA: Lippincott; 1995.
7. National Heart, Lung, and Blood Institute. Expert panel report 2: Guidelines for the Diagnosis and Management of Asthma. July, 1997.
8. Wright SE, Garza CA, Jenkinson SG. Introduction to pulmonary function testing. In: DiPiro JT, Talbert RL, Yee GC, et al., editors. *Pharmacotherapy: A Pathophysiologic Approach*. Stamford, CT: Appleton & Lange; 1997. p.543–52.
9. Jain P, Kavuru MS, Emerman CL, et al. Utility of peak expiratory flow monitoring. *Chest* 1998;114:861–76.
10. Kennedy DT, Chang Z, Small RE. Selection of peak flow meters in ambulatory asthma patients. *Chest* 1998;114:587–92.
11. American Thoracic Society. Standardization of spirometry; 1994 update. *Am J Respir Crit Care Med* 1995;152:1107–36.

Self-Study Questions

Objective
State physical assessment procedures that are routinely conducted for ambulatory care patients with asthma.

1. List the physical assessment procedures routinely conducted for patients with asthma.

Objective
Explain the role of the various types of physical assessment information required for the database of ambulatory care patients with asthma in planning their pharmaceutical care.

2. Explain the role of the expanded respiratory exam in planning the pharmaceutical care of ambulatory care patients with asthma.

3. Explain the role of PFTs in planning the pharmaceutical care of ambulatory care patients with asthma.

4. Explain the importance of height and weight measurements in planning the pharmaceutical care of pediatric ambulatory care patients with asthma.

Objective
Explain factors unique to ambulatory care patients with asthma when interpreting their general appearance.

5. Why is posture an important factor to consider when interpreting the general appearance of a patient with asthma?

6. Why is speech an important factor to consider when interpreting the general appearance of a patient with asthma?

7. Why is level of consciousness an important factor to consider when interpreting the general appearance of a patient with asthma?

Objective
Explain correct technique for using a stethoscope to examine an ambulatory care asthma patient.

8. Describe a technique that may be helpful for getting a pediatric patient to breathe properly during an examination with a stethoscope.

9. Describe the appropriate placement of a stethoscope when auscultating for breath sounds.

10. Describe seven steps important during auscultation of breath sounds with a stethoscope.

Objective
Explain correct technique for the use of a peak flow meter.

11. Describe the steps that should be followed before a patient blows into a peak flow meter.

12. What is the number of times a peak flow measurement should be taken in one session?

13. How is a number chosen for a final recording?

Objective
When given the results of a physical assessment of an ambulatory care patient with asthma, accurately interpret the results.

14. You obtain the following result of a PFT for a patient: FEV_1 69% of predicted value for person of the same age, sex, height, and race. What is your interpretation of this result?

15. Following a dose of a bronchodilator, you obtain the following result for the patient described in question 14: FEV_1 86% of predicted value for person of the same age, sex, and race. What is your interpretation of this result?

16. You obtain the following result of a peak flow meter for a male adult patient: 525 L/min. What is your interpretation of this result?

Self-Study Answers

1. Patients with asthma differ in the physical assessment procedures required for the monitoring and diagnosis of their disease. Physical assessment procedures might include height, weight, blood pressure, pulse, respiratory rate and pattern, evaluation of general appearance, expanded respiratory evaluation with auscultation, and PFT.

2. The expanded respiratory exam is useful in evaluating the current status of the patient with asthma. It can be used to determine whether a significant breathing problem exists as well as to determine response to a rescue medication. It is important to remember that this exam should be part of a comprehensive evaluation that includes a patient history and necessary laboratory findings.

3. PFT should be used in the initial diagnosis of the patient with asthma to determine reversibility of the airway obstruction. In addition, PFT can be followed sequentially (especially with peak flow meters) to determine severity of exacerbation and response to changes in medications.

4. Height and weight should be followed to determine that the patient is growing appropriately. Weight will be necessary for dosing of some medications.

5. Posture may reflect breathing difficulty. Patients may appear hunched over and may resist lying down when they are experiencing breathing difficulty.

6. A patient with asthma conserving energy for breathing may use short phrases or single words rather than entire sentences when speaking.

7. A patient with asthma who is in significant respiratory distress may appear confused and disoriented.

8. Ask the patient to blow out an imaginary flame on the end of your finger.

9. Place the stethoscope on the chest using the diaphragm side of the stethoscope.

10.
    - The patient should lean forward with arms folded to listen across the back.
    - To listen at the anterior chest, the patient should sit erect.
    - The patient will need to be able to take slow, deep breaths through the mouth. You may have to demonstrate for the patient the pace and depth of these breaths.
    - The stethoscope should be placed on the chest using the diaphragm of the stethoscope.
    - Other than the chest excursion, there should be no movement of the patient or the stethoscope while evaluating a breath.
    - You will need to listen in all quadrants of the lung fields.
    - You will need to listen during inspiration and expiration.

11. Be sure that the sliding marker or arrow on the peak flow meter is at the bottom of the numbered scale (at zero or the lowest number on the scale); remove gum or food from the mouth; stand up straight and take as deep a breath as possible. The mouthpiece should be placed into the mouth and the lips closed tightly around the mouthpiece; keep the tongue away from the mouthpiece.

12. 3

13. highest of three measurements

14. These results indicate that mild obstruction to air flow is present.

15. These results indicate that the air flow obstruction is reversible.

16. The obtained reading is within the normal limits reported for peak flows for male patients. This information must be interpreted cautiously, as peak flow readings are most helpful when compared to the patient's best. An isolated peak flow reading must be bundled with all of the other patient parameters to be useful.

Creating a Patient-Specific Database
Part 2: Laboratory Data

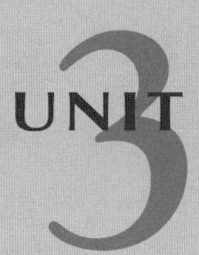
UNIT 3

Unit Objectives	36
Unit Organization	36
Laboratory Tests Used in Ambulatory Care Patients with Asthma	36
Chest X-ray	36
Complete Blood Count	36
Allergy Testing	37
Oxygen Saturation Testing (Pulse Oximetry or Ear Oximetry)	37
The Pharmacist's Role in Laboratory Data Collection	38
Case Study	38
Practice Example	39
Summary	39
References	39
Self-Study Questions	40
Self-Study Answers	41

In unit 2 you learned about performing and interpreting physical assessments of patients with asthma. In this unit you will learn about other objective measures used in the evaluation of patients with asthma. These measures are grouped together as laboratory data.

Many chronic diseases rely heavily on laboratory evaluations for diagnosis and monitoring of disease progression or remission. Asthma is one of the few chronic diseases in which laboratory data is used only occasionally in evaluation of a patient. The decision to obtain laboratory data is based on information gathered during a physical assessment or a history interview. Laboratory data in the assessment of asthma is occasionally used as a component of the diagnosis or for evaluation of specific triggers. Some laboratory information might be used to identify patients in respiratory distress or as part of monitoring medication therapy.

Unit Objectives

After you successfully complete this unit, you will be able to:
- state which laboratory tests are sometimes performed for ambulatory care patients with asthma,
- explain the role of laboratory data when planning the pharmaceutical care of ambulatory care patients with asthma, and
- accurately interpret laboratory test results for ambulatory care patients with asthma.

Unit Organization

For each laboratory test discussed, you will learn its purpose, sources from which you may obtain this data, a description of what the data represents, and how to interpret the results. You will learn which tests the pharmacist can perform and which laboratory data must come from a physician or other source. We will then discuss further the cases of Jeremy Morgan and Mr. Kelley to provide you with practice deciding which laboratory tests might be useful and how to interpret the results of those tests.

Laboratory Tests Used in Ambulatory Care Patients with Asthma

As mentioned in both units 1 and 2, the diagnosis of asthma is multifactorial and relies heavily on the patient's or caregiver's description of symptoms. A physical assessment is used to corroborate interview findings. Laboratory analysis is only occasionally used. Laboratory data may be used in a variety of ways in the treatment of the patient with asthma.

Chest X-ray

Although asthma is a disease of the lungs, a chest X-ray is not often used in evaluation of patients. Most patients with asthma have a normal X-ray. This test is used to rule out other conditions that could be producing similar symptoms or confounding the asthma exacerbation (e.g., infection or foreign body). A chest X-ray is also used with patients not responding well to therapy. If abnormal, the X-ray of a patient with asthma in acute distress will show hyperinflation, consistent with constriction of airways. Chest X-rays are most often obtained when the patient has been hospitalized for an acute exacerbation. The pharmacist may have the results in a discharge summary or in emergency room visit documentation.

Complete Blood Count

A complete blood count (CBC) may be obtained in ambulatory care patients with asthma for several reasons:
- to look for signs of eosinophilia,
- to look for abnormal white blood cell count and differential in patients suspected of having an infectious component to their disease presentation, or
- to check hemoglobin for appropriate oxygen-carrying capacity.

These measures are not useful in every patient, but may be helpful in some cases.

Eosinophilia has been associated with asthma and the degree of eosinophilia has been correlated to asthma severity.[1] Clinically, the presence or absence of eosinophilia does not provide information unattainable from medical history or physical exam. In determining the diagnosis of asthma, the presence of eosinophilia may aid the physician in differentiating asthma from chronic bronchitis.

Viral infections and other respiratory infections can exacerbate a patient's asthma symptoms. Sinusitis has been documented in a large percentage of patients with asthma. Identification and treatment of these upper respiratory tract symptoms is integral to asthma management.[2] An abnormal white blood cell count and differential will aid in identifying an underlying infectious component in an exacerbated state.

Allergy Testing

The identification and subsequent avoidance of known triggers is important in preventing recurrent episodes of asthma flares. Medical history alone is not always sufficient to determine the trigger for a patient with asthma, particularly when the trigger is a perennial indoor allergen. In patients with persistent asthma exposed to perennial indoor allergens, allergy testing is recommended.[2] Allergy testing may also be done on patients with outdoor allergens. Determination of the specific allergen may allow immunotherapy to be initiated in selected patients. In other patients, concrete evidence of the allergy is necessary for them or their parents to initiate necessary environmental modifications.

Allergy testing may be done either by skin testing or in vitro testing.[3] It is not done by the ambulatory care pharmacist, but an understanding of the tests is necessary to interpret results and educate the patient. Scratch testing is done by making a superficial wound in the outermost layer of skin and placing a drop of antigen into the wound. Intradermal testing is done by placing 0.01–0.05 ml of diluted antigen between the layers of skin. The patient is then observed for local inflammation. An in vitro radioallergosorbent test (RAST) is usually reserved for cases in which a specific allergen extract is not available, or in which a patient demonstrates a response to control solutions. A RAST measures specific immunoglobulin E (IgE) levels.[3]

Oxygen Saturation Testing (Pulse Oximetry or Ear Oximetry)

Arterial blood gasses are frequently obtained in patients with asthma in acute care settings such as the emergency room or hospital. In the ambulatory care setting, oxygenation is assessed in patients at risk for hypoxemia using a device known as a pulse oximeter or ear oximeter. This noninvasive test measures the ratio of oxygenated hemoglobin to total hemoglobin (SaO_2) using a light source that passes through tissue. The amount of light absorbed by the oxygen-saturated hemoglobin is measured by a sensor. The sensor reading represents the percentage of hemoglobin that has oxygen attached to it. The reading is an accurate approximation of the oxygen saturation that would be obtained from an arterial blood gas. **Figure 1** depicts the setup of a pulse oximeter.[4]

Follow these steps when performing oximetry[4,5]:
- Explain the procedure to the patient, emphasizing that it is noninvasive and takes only a few minutes.
- Rub the area to be used (fingertip, earlobe, or pinna of the ear) to increase local blood flow.
- Secure the measuring probe or sensor to the area.
- Obtain the reading.

Interpretation of the reading depends on knowledge of the device's limitations. The following may lead to inaccurate results from oximetry[4,5]:
- patient movement,
- abnormal hemoglobin (carboxyhemoglobin),
- presence of intravascular dyes,
- nail polish or nail coverings (when using a finger probe),
- inability to detect saturations <83% with the degree of accuracy possible at higher saturations,
- extreme vasoconstriction, or
- extreme alterations in temperature.

Readings <90% indicate the need for intervention. The patient will require a bronchodilator to aid in improving air exchange. Patients with readings <90% after administration of bronchodilator medication or patients who have other symptoms of significant respiratory distress should be considered for emergent referral. If the patient requires intervention with a bronchodilator, a second oximeter reading can be taken or the oximeter can be left on during administration to provide an indication of improvement. The goal is an oxygen saturation >90%.

There are other laboratory tests that might occasionally be done in the ambulatory care patient with asthma in the course of monitoring drug therapy. The tests are drug specific and will be discussed in unit 9, Designing a Monitoring Plan for Patients with Asthma.

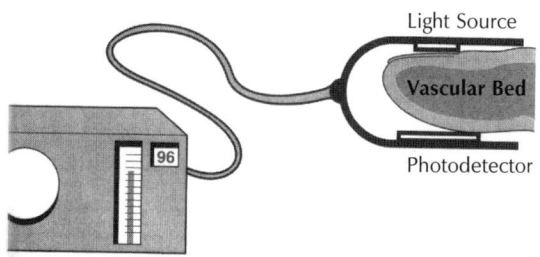

Figure 1. Pulse oximeter setup
Source: reprinted with permission from reference 4.

The Pharmacist's Role in Laboratory Data Collection

Unit 5 of the *Ambulatory Care Clinical Skills Program: Core Module* includes an excellent discussion of sources of laboratory data, including pharmacist-ordered and pharmacist-conducted laboratory tests. Laboratory tests that may be ordered by the pharmacist are more practice specific than disease specific. The majority of the laboratory tests discussed in this unit will not be ordered by the pharmacist. Depending on the practice site, a pharmacist may complete the pulse oximetry and may also draw blood for serum drug concentrations, CBC, or other identified tests. The pharmacist with an ambulatory care asthma practice may choose to maintain an oximetry unit to facilitate patient evaluation and triage. Occupational Safety and Health Administration (OSHA) and the Clinical Laboratory Improvement Amendments of 1988 (CLIA '88) regulations will need to be followed for any laboratory procedure, as described in unit 5 of the *Core Module*.

If you plan to have an oximetry unit available in your practice, it will be important to review the manufacturer's product specifications. These specifications will describe the oximeter's accuracy (the extent to which it agrees with laboratory reference) and precision (the reliability of the test result or the consistency of measurement). You should carefully review the specifications for the probe or sensor to determine whether it is reusable and, if so, how it should be maintained. The manufacturer will also provide instructions for the overall care of the oximetry unit. Although these units are generally easy to care for, their reliability may be compromised if manufacturer guidelines for storage and cleaning are not followed.[5]

Case Study

Now that we've reviewed use of laboratory assessments in the care of ambulatory care patients with asthma, let's return to the case of Jeremy Morgan. As you recall, he is denying that he is in any respiratory distress, although your physical exam contradicts his claim. He does not use a peak flow meter regularly; therefore, you need to use a normal range rather than his personal best for comparison. An oximetry reading might help you evaluate Jeremy. In the meantime, you call Mrs. Morgan at work.

PHARMACIST:
"Mrs. Morgan, I have been collecting additional information about Jeremy's respiratory status while he and I have been talking. I would like to do one more test, if that is OK with you and Jeremy. It is called an oximetry test. I do not have to draw blood, only attach a probe with a light on it to Jeremy's finger for a minute or so. Would that be all right with you?"

MRS. MORGAN:
"He's had that done before in the emergency room. Is there something wrong?"

PHARMACIST:
"It seems to me that Jeremy is working a little harder than he should be to breathe. He may just be nervous. I think this might help us recognize warning signs if he is having difficulty."

MRS. MORGAN:
"Yes. Please, as long as Jeremy is taken care of."

Oximetry results:
March 6, 1999
Oxygen saturation: 89%
Pulse rate: 93

Jeremy's oximeter reading is consistent with your physical findings and reveals that he is in respiratory distress. You will continue with your triage of the situation.

Practice Example

Now it is your turn to practice with Mr. Kelley. He is the middle-aged man that you identified looking at over-the-counter inhalers and who was triaged at his physician's office. He had a stable postbronchodilator physical assessment at your office. He brought with him copies of the interventions done at his physician's office. What laboratory data do you think might have been collected on Mr. Kelley? What additional laboratory data might be planned?

The physician's office drew a CBC with differential to rule out an infectious cause for Mr. Kelley's respiratory distress, but the results were not yet available when Mr. Kelley had left the office. You ask Mr. Kelley to sign a release form for the results when they are available so that your records are complete. You fax the form to the physician's office. The results come back the next morning over your fax machine as follows (normal values are in parentheses):

    Hemoglobin 14 g/dl (14–18 g/dl)
    HCT 41% (39–49%)
    WBC 6000/mm3 (3900–9800/mm^3)
    Differential: Segs 55% (50–70%)
    Bands 2% (3–5%)
    Lymph 23% (20–40%)
    Monos 5% (0–7%)
    Eosinophils 15% (0–5%)

How would you interpret these findings?

The CBC is not indicative of an infectious cause for Mr. Kelley's respiratory distress. That finding is consistent with his description of his symptoms. He has significant eosinophilia that might be a result of the ongoing sensitivity to substances at work.

Mr. Kelley might be a candidate for allergy testing if he continues to have difficulty controlling his symptoms. Identification of the irritant source might be more helpful to the employer than to the overall treatment of your patient.

Summary

In this unit you have been introduced to the laboratory values that may be useful in treating the ambulatory care patient with asthma. You have learned how to use this data along with medical history and physical assessments to provide a snapshot of the patient that can guide therapy decisions. Using the data you have collected in units 2 and 3, you are now prepared to develop a patient-specific database, to be discussed in unit 4.

References

1. O'Connor GT, Weiss ST. Clinical and symptom measures. *Am J Respir Crit Care Med* 1994;149:521–8.
2. National Heart, Lung, and Blood Institute. Expert Panel Report 2: Guidelines for the Diagnosis and Management of Asthma. Bethesda, MD: National Institutes of Health. July, 1997.
3. Demoly P, Michel F-B, Bousquet J. In vivo methods for study of allergy skin test, techniques, and interpretation. In: Middleton E, Ellis E, Yunginger JW, et al., editors. *Allergy: Principles & Practice*, Vol. I. St. Louis, MO: Mosby; 1998. p. 430–9.
4. Pagana KD, Pagana TJ, editors. *Manual of Diagnostic and Laboratory Tests*. St. Louis, MO: Mosby; 1998. p. 1013–16.
5. American Association for Respiratory Care. AARC clinical practice guidelines; pulse oximetry. *Respir Care* 1991;36:1406–9.

Self-Study Questions

Objective
State which laboratory tests are sometimes performed for ambulatory care patients with asthma.

1. List laboratory tests sometimes performed for ambulatory care patients with asthma.

Objective
Explain the role of laboratory data when planning the pharmaceutical care of patients with asthma.

2. What is the role of a CBC when planning the pharmaceutical care of patients with asthma?

3. What is the role of pulse oximetry when planning the pharmaceutical care of patients with asthma?

4. What is the role of allergy testing when planning the pharmaceutical care of patients with asthma?

Objective
Accurately interpret laboratory test results for patients with asthma.

Consider the following case.

Marie Cowling is a 65-year-old widow who has moved to Sun City, AZ, within the last 6 weeks and knows no one in the area. Her two children live in Minneapolis, MN. Marie is a pleasant woman that you have spoken with several times since her arrival. She complains of difficulty maintaining her usual 2-mile-a-day walk. She has been into the pharmacy to refill her Maxair inhaler three times in the past 6 weeks. She moved to the area on the advice of her family physician, Dr. Dobson. Dr. Dobson said the climate change would help Marie's arthritis and breathing problems. Marie returns to your pharmacy today after a visit in the local urgent care facility. At the urgent care facility a CBC was drawn, and she said they placed a red light and probe on the end of her finger. She brings in her discharge papers and asks you to tell her what all the numbers mean. The CBC indicates she had a WBC of 7200/mm^3 with a differential of 2% bands, 85% segs, 13% lymphs. A pulse oximetry reading was noted to be 95%.

5. Interpret the results of her CBC.

6. Interpret the results of her pulse oximetry reading.

Self-Study Answers

1. Patients with asthma do not have routine laboratory tests. Some tests that may be performed on patients with asthma include pulse oximetry, complete blood count, allergy testing, and chest X-ray.

2. The CBC has several components that may assist in the evaluation of the patient with asthma. Your goal should be to optimize oxygenation in patients prone to respiratory distress; therefore, the hemoglobin will help identify those with poor oxygen-carrying capacity. The presence of eosinophilia may corroborate other findings suggesting an allergic component to the presentation of asthma. The WBC and differential will help to identify patients with an infectious etiology for the exacerbation of their symptoms.

3. Pulse oximetry is useful in identifying patients in significant respiratory distress and to monitor improvement after medication administration.

4. Allergy testing may be useful in some patients with asthma to identify their specific triggers and to help formulate a plan for avoiding those substances or modifying the environment to minimize exposure.

5. The CBC is normal.

6. Pulse oximetry is within normal limits.

Creating a Patient-Specific Database
Part 3: Generating the Database

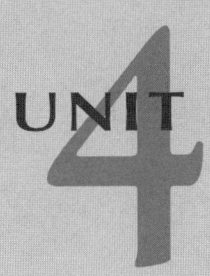

UNIT 4

Unit Objectives	**44**
Unit Organization	**44**
Unique Patient Characteristics That May Affect Interviewing Strategies	**44**
Legal and Ethical Issues	**47**
Case Study	**48**
Practice Example	**49**
Summary	**50**
References	**50**
Self-Study Questions	**51**
Self-Study Answers	**52**
Appendixes	**53**

Using the information you learned in *Ambulatory Care Clinical Skills Program: Core Module* and units 1–3 of this module, you can now answer the question, "How can I generate a patient-specific database that will help me make appropriate therapy decisions?" Maintenance of a patient database mandates that you are aware of legal and ethical issues that arise from collecting confidential patient information. The *Core Module* reviews general legal and ethical concerns that relate to all patients. Patients with asthma will frequently have some additional concerns. Pediatric and adolescent patients may give you confidential information that you will have to decide how to handle. Patients or the parents of patients with asthma may continue smoking despite the negative effects on their disease. In cases of occupational asthma, this information must be kept in the strictest confidence to avoid any possible repercussions in the workplace.

You know how to establish a professional relationship with a patient and find, collect, and generate patient-specific information regarding physical assessment findings and laboratory values. As you have seen, physical assessment findings and laboratory values are not the primary units of evaluation of patients with asthma. A detailed pharmacotherapeutic and health-related history and review of symptoms is necessary to complete the patient database. Using all these tools, you will understand how to generate a patient-specific database for a patient with asthma. You will also be given a chance to practice generating a patient-specific database for a patient with asthma.

Unit Objectives

After you successfully complete this unit, you will be able to:
- identify specific information required for the database that is unique to ambulatory care patients with asthma,
- explain issues unique to ambulatory care patients with asthma when assessing information about them,
- formulate an effective interview strategy to meet the unique needs of ambulatory care patients with asthma,
- explain unique legal and ethical issues that commonly arise in handling the patient-specific information of ambulatory care patients with asthma, and
- generate a patient-specific database for an ambulatory care patient with asthma.

Unit Organization

This unit will begin with a discussion of unique patient characteristics that may affect interviewing strategies. A discussion of the importance of the pharmacotherapeutic and health-related history and review of symptoms follows. Next, a discussion of relevant legal and ethical issues will highlight some important considerations in patients with asthma. Finally, generation of a patient-specific database for ambulatory care patients with asthma will be covered.

Unique Patient Characteristics That May Affect Interviewing Strategies

In the *Core Module* and in unit 1 of this module, you learned there are unique emotional characteristics that need to be addressed in all types of patients. Because asthma affects the entire age range of patients, effective strategies for interviewing patients may differ. Patients with asthma do not always see their breathing difficulties as anything out of the norm. They often accept a degree of respiratory distress as normal. When talking with either asthma patients or their caregiver(s), it is extremely important to ask them about control of their disease and how much medication they require. Remember to ask about technique; have the patient demonstrate inhaler use, when appropriate. Get a clear understanding of the amount of respiratory distress the patient has recently experienced. It is especially important to inquire about nighttime symptoms, which patients may overlook or fail to recognize. You may need to ask a parent or other family member about nighttime symptoms in particular. A checklist of potential patient questions that will prompt you to evaluate these points can be found in **Figure 1**.[1]

In the case of a pediatric or elderly patient, a parent or other caregiver will most likely be needed to help fill in information when gaps exist or the reliability of information is questionable. You will need to recognize that a parent or caregiver may be in control of the medications, but the patient is experiencing the symptoms. A child may be having

Signs and Symptoms/Disease Control

_____ Has your asthma been better or worse since your last visit?

_____ How many times since your last visit have you missed work, school, or a social function because of asthma?

_____ How many times have you needed to go to the emergency room, urgent care facility, or doctor's office since your last visit?

_____ In the past 1–2 weeks, how many times have you:

    ____ woken up at night or had difficulty sleeping because of your asthma symptoms, medications, or coughing?

    ____ had symptoms (wheezing, shortness of breath, coughing, chest tightness) of asthma during the day?

    ____ had symptoms while working or playing?

    ____ needed to use a rescue treatment?

    ____ needed to step up your therapy?

Be sure to ask the patient what changes in activities and environment have taken place since his or her last visit.

Medication Adherence

_____ What medications (prescription, nonprescription, or herbal products) are you currently taking?

_____ How often do you take each medication?

_____ How much medication do you take each time?

_____ We all have trouble remembering to take our medications. How many times in the past 1–2 weeks have you forgotten to take a dose of medication?

_____ Have you had any difficulty filling your prescription?

_____ How many inhalers have you finished in the last month?

_____ Are you experiencing any side effects or unwanted effects from your medications?

Figure 1. Assessment checklist for patient interview
Source: reprinted with permission from reference 1.

significant symptoms, but when you inquire about medication administration the parent may report no need for rescue or as-needed medications. Many parents hesitate when giving their child medications from fear of addiction, fear of overusing the medication and making it ineffective, or inability to assess symptoms. These conflicts exist for caregivers of adult patients as well.

In the *Core Module* you learned several ways to prioritize patients that would be the best candidates for generating a patient database. Obviously, time and economic factors prevent you from creating an extensive database for each patient in your practice. Among asthma patients there is a subset considered at high risk for death from asthma. These patients would certainly benefit from a more structured relationship with you. **Table 1** lists the risk factors for death associated with asthma.[1] Patients with uncontrolled asthma should also be given high priority as you triage patients. Signs and symptoms of poorly controlled asthma include:

- nighttime symptoms,
- need for inhaled $beta_2$-adrenergic agonists several times a day,
- need to refill short-acting $beta_2$-adrenergic agonists more than once a month,
- overuse of long-acting $beta_2$-adrenergic agonists,
- emergency department or urgent care visits due to symptoms,
- nonadherence to inhaled corticosteroid regimen,
- missed school or work, and
- physical activity reduced or symptoms of exercise-induced asthma.

The patient interview is crucial to evaluation of the patient with asthma. As discussed in previous units, asthma is an episodic disease with periods of exacerbation. Between exacerbations, normal status will differ for each patient. The intermittent nature of the disease makes the patient interview an important tool for evaluating overall disease control. During the interview, ask the patient to provide detailed information about only the previous 1–2 weeks. Asking for details beyond this period stretches the patient's ability to recall specific information; ask only general questions about periods beyond 2 weeks. The Life Quality Test designed by the American College of Allergy, Asthma & Immunology (ACAAI) is a simple questionnaire that can be filled out by the patient. This tool will aid in assessment of your patient's

Table 1. Risk Factors for Death Associated with Asthma

Past history of sudden severe exacerbations

Prior intubation for asthma

Prior admissions for asthma to an intensive care unit

Two or more admissions to the hospital for asthma within past 12 months

Three or more emergency care visits for asthma within past 12 months

Hospitalization or emergency care visits for asthma within last month

Use of >2 canisters per month of inhaled short-acting $beta_2$-adrenergic agonists

Current use of or recent withdrawal from systemic corticosteroids

Difficulty perceiving airflow obstruction or its severity

Comorbidity from cardiovascular diseases or chronic obstructive pulmonary disease

Serious psychiatric disease or psychosocial problems

Low socioeconomic status and urban residence

Illicit drug use

Sensitivity to *Alternaria*

Source: reprinted with permission from reference 1.

overall status. An example of this test is available in **Appendix A**.[2]

Legal and Ethical Issues

Legal and ethical issues can arise with any patient encounter. Confidentiality is a major patient concern, reflected in the prominence of legislative agendas that focus on patient rights and confidentiality. Unit 2 of the *Core Module* reviews general information regarding procedures that protect patient confidentiality. The importance of keeping patient-specific information confidential, even if the patient is a minor, has been discussed above. Beyond confidentiality, what other types of issues should be considered?

Both children and adults may abuse illegal substances and use of these substances should be considered in your overall evaluation. The newest trend in adolescent and teenage substance abuse is called "huffing," the inhalation of aerosolized propellants or chemical fumes to get high. This activity can lead to death in any patient; when combined with asthma, the potential mortality is compounded. Reference is frequently made to exposure to tobacco smoke and its impact on the quality of life of patients with asthma. Any substance that is burned and inhaled, even passively, by the patient with asthma can precipitate an exacerbation, including illegal substances such as marijuana as well as incense and fumes from wood-burning fireplaces.

Other situations detrimental to the health of a person with asthma include:
- smoking;
- environmental issues (house dust, cockroaches, and pets); and
- medication issues (inability to administer medications appropriately).

Although exposure to any of these situations can be harmful to either a pediatric or adult patient, pediatric exposure carries with it more significant legal and ethical ramifications, which arise because a parent or caregiver is responsible for the welfare of a child. Adult patients are considered to be responsible for the control of their own environment, but pediatric patients depend on their parents or guardians to provide a safe environment. In some instances, smoking by either parent has placed a child's health at such risk that the child has been removed from the home. Additional issues may arise if parents are not effectively managing and administering a child's medications. In this case, help from social services or a visiting nurse may be required. Parents may be unable to pay for medications or consistently administer prescribed medications to a child. The child's home environment needs to be maintained in a manner that reduces environmental exposures. Parents may require the help of social services with the child's home environment.

Some parents hand over responsibility for medication management to a very young child who is not ready to manage his or her own medications. Ask parents and patients who gives the medication and who is responsible for remembering to take doses. Children mature at different rates and are able to take on responsibility for managing their medications at different ages.

A legal issue to consider in connection with asthma is school truancy. Children with uncontrolled asthma will most likely have high rates of absenteeism; however, as children age, it will be necessary to establish whether the absenteeism is due to truancy or to asthma exacerbations. As a pharmacist, your responsibility is not to correct a truancy issue but to correct the underlying health problem that causes absenteeism. It may be necessary to decide whether a patient is experiencing uncontrolled asthma or merely taking advantage of his or her chronic disease status. Social services can be notified in the case of truancy. Laws vary by state, so you may want to check with your local social service agency about procedures to investigate truancy.

Adult absenteeism can also be a concern. Adults that miss significant amounts of work because of their or their child's illness may be at risk for losing their jobs. Helping patients manage their disease may reduce absenteeism.

As stated earlier, it is important to maintain patient confidentiality in cases of occupational asthma. When counseling a patient with work-related asthma, inform the patient that even general inquiries about the potential adverse effects of work exposures has in some cases resulted in job loss or other employee sanctions.[1] Patients need to be fully aware of this if they decide to approach company management. Many employees do not want their employer to know they have a health problem, much less a chronic disease. Patients may be wary of informing their employer for fear of losing their job or health insurance, even if the precipitating factor is not work related.

Case Study

Using a patient with asthma as an example, we will focus on collecting information in each of the following categories: demographics, medical information, behavioral/lifestyle information, drug therapy, social/economic/quality of life, and personal limitations.

Let's refer back to the case of Jeremy Morgan. **Appendix B** contains a completed Pharmacist's Patient Medical History Form, which both Jeremy and his mother completed, a completed Pharmacist's Patient Database Form, and an Assessment of General Appearance form. Remember that an informed consent signed by Jeremy's mother is necessary because Jeremy is a minor. Jeremy brings the consent and completed Pharmacist's Patient Medical History Form with him to the appointment.

The interview with Jeremy is somewhat jumbled. The pharmacist notes Jeremy is in distress and encourages him to use his albuterol inhaler, giving the pharmacist a perfect opportunity to evaluate Jeremy's inhaler technique. After about 15 minutes, Jeremy's distress resolves. On trying to narrow down what caused his exacerbation, Jeremy and the pharmacist determine that Jeremy's nervousness about coming in for the interview combined with the fact that he ran all the way from school (his mother had to work late) probably precipitated the episode. After Jeremy is feeling better, he agrees to continue with the interview. The fact that the pharmacist was supportive and able to help during Jeremy's exacerbation aids in the formation of a trusting relationship.

Let's review a portion of the interview.

PHARMACIST:
"Jeremy, I'm glad we were able to help you feel better quickly. Do your symptoms occur often?"

JEREMY:
"No, not really. Only when I forget to use my inhaler before I participate in sports. I just wasn't thinking of coming here as a sports activity."

PHARMACIST:
"How about at night? Do you sleep all right?"

JEREMY:
"Sure, I sleep fine."

PHARMACIST:
"Do you need to use any of your medications during the night?"

JEREMY:
"Only when I've got a cold or something and then I just hook up my nebulizer and let it run all night; I sleep in the recliner next to it."

PHARMACIST:
"How often is that?"

JEREMY:
"I guess once every month or so."

PHARMACIST:
"That must be uncomfortable, sleeping in a chair all night."

JEREMY:
"It is, but I already sleep with three pillows to help me breathe. I don't think I can use any more!"

During this part of the interview, you can see how the pharmacist used open-ended questions to dig deeper. The pharmacist uncovered some significant information: It appears Jeremy has continual nighttime symptoms that reflect uncontrolled asthma. Nighttime symptoms are often overlooked. Jeremy demonstrated that he accepts his breathing difficulties as normal and was unable to recognize that his need to run a nebulizer all night and sleep in an elevated position are symptoms of uncontrolled asthma and not recommended therapy. It is important to recognize patients' assumptions about their symptoms and disease.

As we look at the Pharmacist's Patient Database Form, what demographic information is needed? Jeremy's demographic information is important, as is the physician data. You will need a record of Jeremy's age, race, and sex, as all are important information.

About one third of asthma patients are under the age of 18. Uncontrolled asthma in the pediatric population has significant consequences. Asthma is the third leading cause of hospitalization in pediatric patients.[3] More than 10 million lost school days occur annually due to asthma; this is the leading chronic condition to cause school absenteeism.[3] When generating a patient-specific database for a child with asthma, note additional information, such as parental marital status and sibling information. Some of this information can be found on the Pharmacist's Patient Medical History Form. Also, school name and phone number will be helpful as well as whether the school employs a nurse. You may need to communicate with either the school nurse or a designated school representative in the future.

Race is equally important to note. The mortality rate attributed to asthma is significantly higher in the African American population. Occupation is not relevant in Jeremy's case, but occupation can be extremely important in the management of adult patients with asthma. Asthma can affect an employee's ability to perform certain jobs. Asthma-related job absenteeism will be viewed differently, depending on the employer. Identifying patients who may experience occupational asthma depends on the nature of their job.

Jeremy's medical history will be important for evaluating control of his asthma. The number of emergency room visits and hospitalizations will help form a picture of Jeremy's asthma. This number will also be helpful in determining corticosteroid supplementation ("bursts") Jeremy has required in the past year.

The rest of the form contains important information directly related to Jeremy's asthma. In Jeremy's case, there is a note that he experiences difficulty participating in gym class and had to quit the cross-county track team last spring. There is also a difference between the patient form and the pharmacist form that can be noted in the alcohol and tobacco use sections. The form filled out by Jeremy and his mother indicates that Jeremy does not use alcohol or tobacco. However, during the interview, Jeremy cautiously told the pharmacist that he and his buddies have experimented with both cigarettes and beer in the past couple of months. Although this discrepancy presents a tricky situation, it is not unusual. As a pharmacist, you need to remember that information is confidential between you and your patient. A breach of that trust, even if it were in the interest of his health, would be unethical. The pharmacist's role should be to encourage Jeremy to avoid alcohol and tobacco, especially with his asthma. The pharmacist assured Jeremy that his parents would not be told, and the pharmacist encouraged Jeremy to discuss his experimentation with his parents. Do not forget to inquire about environment (pets, triggers in the home, and cleanliness) and ability to pay for medications and note the information in the Family/Social/Economic Section. Jeremy does not have any concerns in these areas, but these issues arise with many patients with asthma.

The laboratory data has been filled in. A peak flow meter reading was completed just before Jeremy left the pharmacist's office.

On demonstration, Jeremy's inhaler technique was good and he had an excellent response to his rescue therapy. The pharmacist made a few notations about adherence to therapy regimen and noted the nighttime nebulizer use. The pharmacist also noted periodic use of ibuprofen for fevers associated with colds and the nutritional supplements that Jeremy takes. Although his vaccines are up to date, he has never received an influenza vaccine. The pharmacist will make a note to have Jeremy receive a vaccine in the fall. With pediatric patients, evaluating vaccine history is especially important. In general, vaccination rates in the United States continue to be less than ideal.

Practice Example

Now that we have covered some legal and ethical issues surrounding asthma management, let's take a look at the case of Mr. Kelley. Drawing on the information you learned in units 1–3 and the completed Pharmacist's Patient Medical History Form in **Appendix C**, use the blank Pharmacist's Patient Database Form and Assessment of General Appearance form supplied in Appendix C to fill in information we decided to gather. When you are finished, compare your completed form to the one in **Appendix D**. If you find gaps in information, go back to the corresponding section in this unit or to unit 6 of the *Core Module*.

Turn to the completed Pharmacist's Patient Database Form in Appendix D. As you can see, there are entries for the original date the pharmacist interacted with Mr. Kelley (May 5, 1999) and an update when he returned to the pharmacy (June 12, 1999).

Mr. Kelley is a 43-year-old white male with a childhood history of asthma. He also has a 5-year history of hypertension, for which he receives hydrochlorothiazide 25 mg each day. He has a family history of cardiac disease: father and brother have had myocardial infarctions. His mother has type 2 diabetes.

Mr. Kelley has been diagnosed with occupational asthma per his recent physician visit. He has also experienced exacerbations outside of work that may have been precipitated by his work-related exposure. It will be important to monitor these symptoms to determine if he continues to have difficulties outside of work. Mr. Kelley's medical condition is further complicated by hypertension and two risk factors for coronary heart disease.

Mr. Kelley coaches his son's soccer team and frequently plays basketball with the neighborhood men. He does not smoke and drinks one or two beers per week.

Aside from his hydrochlorothiazide, Mr. Kelley did not routinely take any medications until onset of his asthma. He occasionally takes ibuprofen after neighborhood basketball games.

Mr. Kelley is up to date for all preventive health measures and routine vaccinations. He does not usually get an influenza vaccine.

Summary

Regardless of the documentation method you select, it should include the basic elements outlined in this unit. Always take care to be consistent with your documentation and be mindful of any legal or ethical issues that may arise. Patient confidentiality should always be stressed. Spending a few extra minutes to keep digging to get more accurate answers to your questions will benefit the patient and can be used to refine the treatment plan to best meet patient needs and goals.

References

1. National Heart, Lung, and Blood Institute. Expert Panel Report 2: Guidelines for the Diagnosis and Management of Asthma. July 1997.
2. American College of Allergy, Asthma & Immunology (ACAAI) website, accessed June 1999. (http://allergy.mcg.edu/lifequality/index.html)
3. American Lung Association. American Lung Association Fact Sheet: Asthma in Children. Available at: www.lungusa.org, accessed January 4, 1999.

Self-Study Questions

Objective
Identify specific information required for the database that is unique to ambulatory care patients with asthma.

1. List specific information unique to ambulatory care patients with asthma required to address their health care needs and to make appropriate pharmacotherapeutic and health-related decisions and recommendations.

Objective
Explain issues unique to ambulatory care patients with asthma when assessing information about them.

2. Why is the presence or absence of nighttime symptoms an issue when assessing information about patients with asthma?

3. Why is the refill history of short-acting $beta_2$-adrenergic agonists an issue when assessing information about patients with asthma?

4. Why is information about recent hospital admissions or intensive care unit admissions an issue when assessing information about patients with asthma?

Objective
Formulate an effective interview strategy to meet the unique needs of ambulatory care patients with asthma.

5. Describe effective interview strategies for meeting the unique needs of ambulatory care patients with asthma.

Objective
Explain unique legal and ethical issues that commonly arise in handling the patient-specific information of patients with asthma.

6. Name and explain a unique legal issue that arises in handling patient-specific information of patients with asthma.

7. Name and explain a unique ethical issue that commonly arises in handling a patient with asthma.

8. Explain why confidentiality of patient-specific information in cases of occupational asthma is extremely important.

Objective
Generate a patient-specific database for an ambulatory care patient with asthma.

9. Refer to the case of Marie Cowling as described in unit 3. Refer to her completed Pharmacist's Patient Medical History Form in **Appendix E**. Using this information, complete the blank Pharmacist's Patient Database Form supplied in Appendix E to fill in the pieces of information available.

Self-Study Answers

1. You need to know types of daily activities for scheduling medications, living environment, triggers, nighttime symptoms, work environment (triggers), health benefit, health care beliefs, concerns about long-term use of medications, person responsible for medication administration, number of exacerbations, and quality of life factors.

2. Many patients may not recognize nighttime coughing as a symptom of poorly controlled asthma.

3. Frequent use or overuse of a short-acting $beta_2$-adrenergic agonists is a sign of uncontrolled asthma. Adherence or inappropriate therapy may be an issue.

4. Patients with hospital admissions, especially to the intensive care unit, are at risk for death due to asthma.

5. Unique interview strategies include speaking with both the patient and the caregiver. Assessing quality of life issues and determining how to best meet the needs of a patient with asthma (scheduling, school, work, and physical activities) will be essential.

6. Child endangerment from inappropriate living conditions, smoking in the home, or poor medication administration in the case of pediatric patients with asthma may result in legal actions against the parent or caregiver.

7. Pediatric patients may divulge to you that they have used alcohol, tobacco, or an illegal substance. This information must be kept confidential and not shared with the child's parents.

8. In some instances, inquires about occupational asthma and the effects of the workplace may place the employee at risk for losing their job or health insurance.

9. When you are finished compare your form to the completed form in **Appendix F**. If you find gaps in any information, go back to the corresponding section in this unit or unit 6 of the *Core Module*.

Welcome to the Life Quality Test

If you or your child has been told you have asthma, or even if you have occasional problems taking a good, deep breath, this simple test from the American College of Allergy, Asthma & Immunology (ACAAI) may help improve your LIFE QUALITY (or "LQ"). Just answer these 20 questions and decide whether a quick, free phone call could lead to a better LQ for you.

ACTIVITIES

When I walk or do simple chores, I have trouble breathing or I cough.	Yes	No
When I perform heavier work, such as walking up hills and stairs or doing chores that involve lifting, I have trouble breathing or I cough.	Yes	No
Sometimes I avoid exercising or taking part in sports like jogging, swimming, tennis or aerobics because I have trouble breathing or I cough.	Yes	No
I have been unable to sleep through the night without coughing attacks or shortness of breath.	Yes	No

SYMPTOMS

Sometimes I can't catch a good, deep breath.	Yes	No
Sometimes I make wheezing sounds in my chest.	Yes	No
Sometimes my chest feels tight.	Yes	No
Sometimes I cough a lot.	Yes	No

TRIGGERS

Dust, pollen and pets make my asthma, cough or trouble breathing worse.	Yes	No
My asthma gets worse in cold weather.	Yes	No
My asthma gets worse and worse when I'm around tobacco smoke, fumes or strong odors.	Yes	No
When I catch a cold it often goes to my chest.	Yes	No

HOSPITAL VISITS

I made one or more emergency visits due to asthma or breathing problems in the last year.	Yes	No
I had one or more overnight hospitalizations due to asthma or breathing problems in the last year.	Yes	No

MEDICATION PROBLEMS

I feel like I use my asthma inhaler too often.	Yes	No
Sometimes I don't like the way my asthma medicine(s) make me feel.	Yes	No
My asthma medicine doesn't control my asthma.	Yes	No

ANXIETIES

My breathing problem or asthma controls my life more than I would like.	Yes	No
I feel tension or stress because of my breathing problem or asthma.	Yes	No
I worry that my breathing problem or asthma affects my health or may even shorten my life.	Yes	No

If you answered "yes" to one or more questions on this test, you may be able to reduce your asthma symptoms and improve your life quality. An allergist can help you.

Take these steps now:
- Continue your present asthma treatment until you've consulted your doctor.
- If you have an allergist, schedule an appointment as soon as possible.
- Discuss this LQ Test with your doctor.

Source: reference 2.

APPENDIX B

Patient Consent and Release Statement

I understand that my Breathe Rite Pharmacy Care Center pharmacist will be working to help me improve and maintain my health through a better understanding of my health problems and helping me make the most effective use of my medications. As part of this process, Breathe Rite Pharmacy Care Center will provide health-related information about me and the services I have received to my physicians to keep them informed of my progress.

I hereby authorize Breathe Rite Pharmacy Care Center to release to my physician all information and records related to the care I receive.

I understand that a portion of the service includes my giving a series of blood samples for the purpose of monitoring. There may be some discomfort, bruising, bleeding, or swelling at the puncture site and surrounding tissue, and it may become infected. If signs of infection are seen (redness, swelling, warmth, pain, or pus), I will seek medical care from my physician.

I hereby release Breathe Rite Pharmacy Care Center, their affiliates, directors, officers, employees, successors, and assigns from any and all liability arising from or in any way connected with such release of such information and with this blood drawing for my measurements. I understand that I should not participate in these tests if I suffer from any bleeding disorder or similar condition.

Date: __3/2/99__

Patient Printed Name: __Jeremy Morgan__

Patient or Guardian Signature: __Sally Morgan__

Pharmacist's Patient Medical History Form

I. Patient Information

Name: **Jeremy Morgan**

Address: **128 Water Ave   Milford, IL   60243**

Home Phone: **222-2222**   Office Phone: _____

Date of Birth: **1-13-86**   Last year of education completed: **7th grade**

Patient lives with **Parents + sister + brother**

Caregiver (if applicable): **N/A**

Caregiver Phone: _____

Employer: **N/A**   Job Title: _____

Name of Health Insurer: **Healthy Day**

Health Ins. Card #: **11-111-111-1-03**   Social Security #: **222-22-2222**

Primary Care Physician's Name: **Dr. Lefton**   Phone: **222-3111**

Specialist Physician's Name: _____   Phone: _____

Other Health Care Practitioner: _____   Phone: _____

II. Medical History

Are you allergic to any prescription drugs or over-the-counter medications? _____
☐ Yes   ☒ No   If yes, please list the medications and type of allergic reaction experienced:

_____

Are there any medications that you are not allergic to but cannot tolerate? _____
☐ Yes   ☒ No   If yes, please list the medications and the reaction experienced:

_____

Do you use tobacco?
☐ Yes   ☒ No   If yes, what type? _____   How often? _____

Do you drink alcohol?
☐ Yes   ☒ No   If yes, what type? _____   How often? _____

Name: _Jeremy Morgan_

Please put a check (✔) next to those items listed below that apply to you:

HEART PROBLEMS	✔	URINARY/REPRODUCTIVE	✔
Chest pain (angina)		Urinary or bladder infection	
Past heart attack		Prostate problems	
Heart failure		Hysterectomy	
Irregular heartbeat		Chronic yeast infections	
Heart by-pass surgery		Kidney disease	
Rheumatic fever		Dialysis	
Other:		Other:	

EYES, EARS, NOSE & THROAT	✔	MUSCLES AND BONES	✔
Poor vision		Arthritis	
Poor hearing		Gout	
Glaucoma		Back problems	
Sinus problems		Amputation	
Balance disorder		Joint replacement	
Other:		Other:	

GASTROINTESTINAL	✔	NEUROLOGICAL	✔
Heartburn		Headaches	
Ulcer		Seizures or epilepsy	
Constipation		Parkinson's disease	
Diverticulitis		Dizziness	
Liver disease		Past stroke	
Gallbladder problems		Fainting	
Pancreatitis		Depression	
Other:		Anxiety	
		Other:	

DO YOU HAVE:	✔	LUNG PROBLEMS	✔
High blood pressure		Asthma	✓
Low blood pressure		Emphysema	
High cholesterol		Bronchitis	
Diabetes		Other:	
Cancer			
Anemia			
Bleeding disorder		**DO YOU HAVE OR USE …?**	✔
Hay fever		Glasses	✓
Sleeping problems		Hearing aid	
Other:		Other:	

DO YOU HAVE A FAMILY HISTORY OF:			
High blood pressure		Asthma	✓
Heart disease	✓	Other:	
Diabetes			

Name: _Jeremy Morgan_

III. CURRENT PRESCRIPTION MEDICATIONS (INCLUDING ONES RECEIVED AT OTHER PHARMACIES)

Name of prescription medicine and strength (i.e., milligrams, grams, and units)	How much do you take each time?	How many times a day do you take the medicine?	Medical problem being treated	When did you start taking this medicine?	Has the medicine helped you? Yes/No	Name of doctor or specialist who prescribed the medicine
Example: Diabeta, 2.5 mg	1	2	Diabetes	1992	Yes	Dr. Harold Smith
Azmacort	8 puffs	4 times	asthma	last year	no	Lefton
Albuterol	2 puffs	when I need it	asthma	years ago	yes	Lefton
Albuterol neb. solution	don't know	at night	asthma	years ago	yes	Lefton

IV. CURRENT NONPRESCRIPTION MEDICATIONS

EX: ANTACIDS, ANTI-DIARRHEALS, ALLERGY MEDICINES, ANTI-NAUSEA, DIET PILLS, EAR OR EYE MEDICATIONS, LAXATIVES, PAIN RELIEVERS, VITAMINS, ETC.

Name of medicine Example: Tylenol	How often do you take it? (daily, once a week, etc.)	Name of medicine	How often do you take it?
	for colds		
Motrin IB	daily		
Echinacea	daily		
Vitamin C			

I certify this information is accurate and complete to the best of my knowledge. _Jeremy Morgan_ _3/2/99_
　　　signature　　　　date

© 2000, American Society of Health-System Pharmacists, Inc. All rights reserved.

Appendix B   57

Ambulatory Care Clinical Skills Program: Asthma Management — Appendix B

Original Date: 3/6/99
Date updated: _____
Date updated: _____
Date updated: _____

Pharmacist's Patient Database Form

Demographic and Administrative Information

- **Name:** Jeremy Morgan
- **Social Security #:** 222-22-2222
- **Address:** 123 Water Ave. Milford, IL 60243
- **Health Care Provider's Name:** Dr. Lefton
- **Health Care Provider's Phone:** 222-3111
- **Work Phone:**
- **Home Phone:** 222-2222
- **Date of Birth:** 1-13-86
- **Race:** White
- **Gender:** M
- **Religion:**
- **Occupation:** Child (Mom = Sally)
- **Health Insurer:** Healthy Day
- **Subscriber #:** 11-111-111-1-03
- **Primary Card Holder:** George Morgan
- **Drug Benefit:** ☒ yes ☐ no   copay: $5.00-Generic $10-Brand

Current Symptoms

Wheezing - hx of severe exacerbations & ER visits ↑ in frequency

Past Medical History

- Asthma - diagnosed @ 3 yrs
- 6 ER visits in past 12 mos.
- 4 corticosteroid bursts in 8 months

Acute and Current Medical Problems

1.
2.
3.
4.
5.
6.
7.
8.

Family/Social/Economic History

- ∅ pets ∅ smoking in home
- 2 sibs 8 yr ♀, 5 yr ♂

Cost of medications per month: $ 20.00

Personal Limitations

*Quit cross country team 2° asthma

Allergies/Intolerances

☒ No known drug allergies

Medication	Reaction

Social Drug Use

- **Alcohol:** Experimenting x2 mos.
- **Caffeine:** 2 cokes/day
- **Tobacco:** Experimenting x2 mos.

Pregnancy/Breastfeeding Status

☐ Pregnant (due _____)   ☐ Breastfeeding

Diet

- ☐ Low salt — No
- ☐ Low fat — No
- ☐ Diabetic — No
- Timing of meals:

Routine Exercise/Recreation

Daily Activities/Timing

- school
- play c̄ friends
- roller blade
- bike ride

© 2000, American Society of Health-System Pharmacists, Inc. All rights reserved.

Patient Name: Jeremy Morgan

Physical Assessment/Laboratory Data—Initial/Follow-up

Date	3/6/99				
Height					
Weight	95 lbs				
Temp					
BP					
Pulse	90				
Respirations	24 (shallow)				
Peak Flow	425 l/min				
FBG					
R. Glucose					
HbA_{1c}					
T. Chol.					
LDL					
HDL					
TG					
INR					
BUN					
Cr					
ALT					
AST					
Alk Phos					
Pulse Ox	86% sat/93 pulse				

Drug Serum Concentrations

Date					

Notes:
3/6/99 – use of accessory muscles and wheezing noted on auscultation

Patient Name: Jeremy Morgan

Current Prescription Medication Regimen

Name/Dose/Strength/Route	Schedule/Frequency of Use	Indication	Start Date (and Stop Date If Applicable)	Prescriber	Adherence Issues/Efficacy
Azmacort	8 puffs QID	Asthma	May 1998	Lefton	*poor refill history
Proventil inhaler	2 puffs QID prn	Asthma	years	Lefton	*uses as needed
Proventil Nebs	0.3 ml prn	Asthma	years	Lefton	*frequently uses all night

Current Nonprescription Medication Regimen (OTC, herbal, homeopathic, nutritional, etc.)

Name/Dose/Strength/Route	Schedule/Frequency of Use	Indication	Start Date (and Stop Date If Applicable)	Prescriber	Adherence Issues/Efficacy
Motrin 200 mg	prn	Fever 2° "colds"	?	Self	
Echinacea extract	2 mL Q Day	immune booster	>1 yr	Mom	
Vitamin C 500 mg	2 tablets Q Day	immune booster	>3 yrs	Mom	

©2000, American Society of Health-System Pharmacists, Inc. All rights reserved.

Patient Name: Jeremy Morgan

Risk Assessment/Preventive Measures/Quality of Life

Cardiovascular Risk Assessment			
male >45 years old		1	
female >55 years old or female <55 with history of ovarectomy not taking estrogen replacement		1	
Definite MI or sudden death before age 55 year in father or male first-degree relative or before 65 year in mother or female first-degree relative	N/A	1	
current cigarette smoking		1	
hypertension		1	
diabetes mellitus		1	
HDL cholesterol <35 mg/dl		1	
HDL cholesterol >60 mg/dl		-1	
		Total:	

Is patient at risk for complications of current conditions? ❑ Yes ☒ No
Specify: Mortality 2° to asthma exacerbation

Preventive Measures for Adults H = has been done R = patient refuses X = not applicable		Date			
Women					
Pap Smear/pelvic	Annually 19+				
Mammogram	Every 1-2Y 40-49; annually 50+				
Men					
Rectal/prostate	Annually 50+				
All Patients					
Total/HDL-C	Every 5Y 19+				
Home Fecal Occult Blood Test	Annually				
Immunizations					
Td	Every 10Y	H			
Influenza	Every fall*	Not done			
Pneumovax	Once*	Not done			

* if indicated

Quality of life issues

*childhood vaccines up to date
*Jeremy quit cross-country team 2° to asthma

© 2000, American Society of Health-System Pharmacists, Inc. All rights reserved.

Assessment of General Appearance

Patient __Jeremy Morgan__　　　　　　　　　　　　　Date __3/6/99__

General Appearance	Observations and Comments
Level of consciousness 　alertness: alert, confused, 　delirious, stuporous, comatose, 　orientation: person, place, time	Alert & oriented x3
Signs of distress 　respiratory distress, pain, anxiety, etc.	Difficulty completing sentences
Posture, motor activity, and gait 　*Describe*	Normal posture & gait
Dress, grooming, and personal hygiene 　*Describe*	Normal for a teenager
Affect 　normal, inappropriate 　*Describe*	Quiet - slightly nervous fidgety
Speech 　normal, impaired 　*Describe*	Single word phrases
Skin 　color: normal, blue, brown, red, pallor 　texture: normal, coarse, dry, oily 　turgor: good, poor 　edema 　lesions: color, type, configuration, anatomic 　　distribution, consistency	Pale No skin abnormalities

Pharmacist's Patient Medical History Form

I. Patient Information

Name: **Mike Kelley**
Address: **211 Clear St. Adington, IL**
Home Phone: **111-2345**   Office Phone: **112-3456**
Date of Birth: **1-20-56**   Last year of education completed: **12th grade**
Patient lives with **spouse, 4 children (1 yr, 6 yr, 8 yr, 12 yr)**
Caregiver (if applicable): **N/A**
Caregiver Phone: **N/A**
Employer: **ACME Chemical**   Job Title: **Time Study Coordinator**
Name of Health Insurer: **Catastrophy Plan**
Health Ins. Card #: **911-911-91101**   Social Security #: **333-33-3333**
Primary Care Physician's Name: **Dr. Thompson**   Phone: **911-9111**
Specialist Physician's Name: **N/A**   Phone: ____
Other Health Care Practitioner: **N/A**   Phone: ____

II. Medical History

Are you allergic to any prescription drugs or over-the-counter medications? ____
☒ Yes   ☐ No   If yes, please list the medications and type of allergic reaction experienced:

ASA: face swelling, difficulty breathing

Are there any medications that you are not allergic to but cannot tolerate? ____
☐ Yes   ☒ No   If yes, please list the medications and the reaction experienced:

____

Do you use tobacco?   **smoked from 18 yrs-20 yrs (1/2 pack a day)**
☐ Yes   ☒ No   If yes, what type? ____   How often? ____

Do you drink alcohol?
☒ Yes   ☐ No   If yes, what type? **beer**   How often? **1-2 times a week**

Name: _Mike Kelley_

Please put a check (✔) next to those items listed below that apply to you:

HEART PROBLEMS	✔	URINARY/REPRODUCTIVE	✔
Chest pain (angina)		Urinary or bladder infection	
Past heart attack		Prostate problems	
Heart failure		Hysterectomy	
Irregular heartbeat		Chronic yeast infections	
Heart by-pass surgery		Kidney disease	
Rheumatic fever		Dialysis	
Other:		Other:	

EYES, EARS, NOSE & THROAT	✔	MUSCLES AND BONES	✔
Poor vision		Arthritis	
Poor hearing		Gout	
Glaucoma		Back problems	
Sinus problems		Amputation	
Balance disorder		Joint replacement	
Other:		Other:	

GASTROINTESTINAL	✔	NEUROLOGICAL	✔
Heartburn		Headaches	
Ulcer		Seizures or epilepsy	
Constipation		Parkinson's disease	
Diverticulitis		Dizziness	
Liver disease		Past stroke	
Gallbladder problems		Fainting	
Pancreatitis		Depression	
Other:		Anxiety	
		Other:	

DO YOU HAVE:	✔	LUNG PROBLEMS	✔
High blood pressure	✓	Asthma	✓
Low blood pressure		Emphysema	
High cholesterol		Bronchitis	
Diabetes		Other:	
Cancer			
Anemia			
Bleeding disorder		**DO YOU HAVE OR USE …?**	✔
Hay fever		Glasses	
Sleeping problems		Hearing aid	
Other:		Other:	

DO YOU HAVE A FAMILY HISTORY OF:			
High blood pressure	✓	Asthma	✓
Heart disease	✓	Other:	
Diabetes	✓		

Appendix C 65

Name: _Mike Kelley_

III. Current Prescription Medications (Including ones received at other pharmacies)

Name of prescription medicine and strength (i.e., milligrams, grams, and units)	How much do you take each time?	How many times a day do you take the medicine?	Medical problem being treated	When did you start taking this medicine?	Has the medicine helped you? Yes/No	Name of doctor or specialist who prescribed the medicine
Example: Diabeta, 2.5 mg	1	2	Diabetes	1992	Yes	Dr. Harold Smith
Hydrochlorothiazide 25 mg	1	one	Blood Pressure	5 yrs	yes	Dr. Thompson

IV. Current Nonprescription Medications

Ex: ANTACIDS, ANTI-DIARRHEALS, ALLERGY MEDICINES, ANTI-NAUSEA, DIET PILLS, EAR OR EYE MEDICATIONS, LAXATIVES, PAIN RELIEVERS, VITAMINS, ETC.

Name of medicine Example: Tylenol	How often do you take it? (daily, once a week, etc.)	Name of medicine	How often do you take it?
ibuprofen 200 mg	once-twice/month		

I certify this information is accurate and complete to the best of my knowledge. _Mike Kelley_ _5/5/99_
                                                                                         signature   date

© 2000, American Society of Health-System Pharmacists, Inc. All rights reserved.

Pharmacist's Patient Database Form

Original Date:_____
Date updated:_____
Date updated:_____
Date updated:_____

Demographic and Administrative Information

Name:	Social Security #:
Address:	
Health Care Provider's Name	Health Care Provider's Phone
Work Phone: Home Phone:	Date of Birth:
Race:	Gender:
Religion:	Occupation:
Health Insurer:	Subscriber #:
Primary Card Holder:	Drug Benefit: ❏ yes ❏ no copay: $_____

Current Symptoms

Past Medical History	Acute and Current Medical Problems
	1.
	2.
	3.
	4.
	5.
	6.
	7.
	8.

Family/Social/Economic History	Personal Limitations

Cost of medications per month $_____

Allergies/Intolerances	Social Drug Use
❏ No known drug allergies	Alcohol
Medication Reaction	Caffeine
	Tobacco
	Pregnancy/Breastfeeding Status
	❏ Pregnant (due _____) ❏ Breastfeeding

Diet	Routine Exercise/Recreation	Daily Activities/Timing
❏ Low salt		
❏ Low fat		
❏ Diabetic		
Timing of meals:		

© 2000, American Society of Health-System Pharmacists, Inc. All rights reserved.

Patient Name: _____

Physical Assessment/Laboratory Data—Initial/Follow-up					
Date					
Height					
Weight					
Temp					
BP					
Pulse					
Respirations					
Peak Flow					
FBG					
R. Glucose					
HbA_{1c}					
T. Chol.					
LDL					
HDL					
TG					
INR					
BUN					
Cr					
ALT					
AST					
Alk Phos					

Drug Serum Concentrations

Date					

Notes:

© 2000, American Society of Health-System Pharmacists, Inc. All rights reserved.

Patient Name: _____

Current Prescription Medication Regimen

Name/Dose/Strength/Route	Schedule/Frequency of Use	Indication	Start Date (and Stop Date If Applicable)	Prescriber	Adherence Issues/Efficacy

Current Nonprescription Medication Regimen (OTC, herbal, homeopathic, nutritional, etc.)

Name/Dose/Strength/Route	Schedule/Frequency of Use	Indication	Start Date (and Stop Date If Applicable)	Prescriber	Adherence Issues/Efficacy

©2000, American Society of Health-System Pharmacists, Inc. All rights reserved.

Patient Name: _____

Risk Assessment/Preventive Measures/Quality of Life

Cardiovascular Risk Assessment		
male >45 years old	1	
female >55 years old or female <55 with history of ovarectomy not taking estrogen replacement	1	
Definite MI or sudden death before age 55 year in father or male first-degree relative or before 65 year in mother or female first-degree relative	1	
current cigarette smoking	1	
hypertension	1	
diabetes mellitus	1	
HDL cholesterol <35 mg/dl	1	
HDL cholesterol >60 mg/dl	-1	
	Total:	

Is patient at risk for complications of current conditions? ❏ Yes ❏ No
Specify:

Preventive Measures for Adults H = has been done R = patient refuses X = not applicable		Date				
Women						
Pap Smear/pelvic	Annually 19+					
Mammogram	Every 1-2Y 40-49; annually 50+					
Men						
Rectal/prostate	Annually 50+					
All Patients						
Total/HDL-C	Every 5Y 19+					
Home Fecal Occult Blood Test	Annually					
Immunizations						
Td	Every 10Y					
Influenza	Every fall*					
Pneumovax	Once*					

* if indicated

Quality of life issues

© 2000, American Society of Health-System Pharmacists, Inc. All rights reserved.

Assessment of General Appearance

Patient _____ Date _____

General Appearance	Observations and Comments

Level of consciousness
    alertness: alert, confused, delirious, stuporous, comatose,
    orientation: person, place, time	

Signs of distress respiratory distress, pain, anxiety, etc.	
Posture, motor activity, and gait *Describe*	
Dress, grooming, and personal hygiene *Describe*	

Affect
    normal, inappropriate
    Describe	

Speech
    normal, impaired
    Describe	

Skin
    color: normal, blue, brown, red, pallor
    texture: normal, coarse, dry, oily
    turgor: good, poor
    edema
    lesions: color, type, configuration, anatomic distribution, consistency	

Appendix D 71

Pharmacist's Patient Database Form

Original Date: **5/5/99**
Date updated: _____
Date updated: _____
Date updated: _____

Demographic and Administrative Information

Name: Mike Kelley	Social Security #: 333-33-3333
Address: 211 Clear Street Adington, IL 43430	
Health Care Provider's Name: Dr. Thompson	Health Care Provider's Phone: 911-9111
Work Phone: 112-3456 Home Phone: 111-2345	Date of Birth: 1-20-56
Race: Black	Gender: M
Religion:	Occupation: Time Study Coordinator ACME Chemical
Health Insurer: Catastrophy Plan	Subscriber #: 911-911-91101
Primary Card Holder: Mike Kelley	Drug Benefit: ☐ yes ☒ no copay: $ _____

Current Symptoms

wheezing @ work (X) 1 month

Past Medical History	Acute and Current Medical Problems
asthma as a child	1. Hypertension
	2. Asthma
	3.
	4.
	5.
	6.
	7.
	8.

Family/Social/Economic History	Personal Limitations
Married c̄ 4 children father and brother had M.I. @ 51 yrs and 48 yrs mother has DM	

Cost of medications per month $ _____

Allergies/Intolerances	Social Drug Use
☐ No known drug allergies	Alcohol 1-2x/week (beer)
Medication Reaction	Caffeine
ASA difficulty breathing, face swells	Tobacco not currently
	Pregnancy/Breastfeeding Status
	☐ Pregnant (due _____) ☐ Breastfeeding

Diet	Routine Exercise/Recreation	Daily Activities/Timing
☐ Low salt		
☐ Low fat		
☐ Diabetic		
Timing of meals:		

© 2000, American Society of Health-System Pharmacists, Inc. All rights reserved.

Ambulatory Care Clinical Skills Program: Asthma Management — Appendix D

Patient Name: **Mike Kelley**

Physical Assessment/Laboratory Data—Initial/Follow-up

	*MD office	*Pharmacy			
Date	May 5, 1999	May 5, 1999	June 12, 1999		
Height	5'10"		5'10"		
Weight	186 lbs		184 lbs		
Temp					
BP	130/80 mmHg		128/85 mmHg		
Pulse	78	80	75		
Respirations	20 wheezing shallow	15 and comfortable	15 and comfortable		
Peak Flow					
FBG					
R. Glucose					
HbA$_{1c}$					
T. Chol.					
LDL					
HDL					
TG					
INR					
BUN					
Cr					
ALT					
AST					
Alk Phos					
Hg	14				
HCT	41				
WBC	6.0				
Diff	55^S 28^B 23^L 5^M 15^E				

Drug Serum Concentrations

Date					

Notes: 5/5/98 - exam post albuterol; only occ. wheezes noted
6/12/98 - pt reports improvement c̄ meds

© 2000, American Society of Health-System Pharmacists, Inc. All rights reserved.

Patient Name: Mike Kelley

Current Prescription Medication Regimen

Name/Dose/Strength/Route	Schedule/Frequency of Use	Indication	Start Date (and Stop Date If Applicable)	Prescriber	Adherence Issues/Efficacy
Hydroclorothiazide 25 mg	1 po Q AM	HTN	x 5 yrs	Thompson	good - adherence

Current Nonprescription Medication Regimen (OTC, herbal, homeopathic, nutritional, etc.)

Name/Dose/Strength/Route	Schedule/Frequency of Use	Indication	Start Date (and Stop Date If Applicable)	Prescriber	Adherence Issues/Efficacy
ibuprofen 200 mg	200-400 mg prn	Muscle sore	2 years	-	works well

©2000, American Society of Health-System Pharmacists, Inc. All rights reserved.

74 Ambulatory Care Clinical Skills Program: Asthma Management   Appendix D

Patient Name: __Mike Kelley__

Risk Assessment/Preventive Measures/Quality of Life

Cardiovascular Risk Assessment		
male >45 years old	1	
female >55 years old or female <55 with history of ovarectomy not taking estrogen replacement	1	
Definite MI or sudden death before age 55 year in father or male first-degree relative or before 65 year in mother or female first-degree relative	1	1
current cigarette smoking	1	
hypertension	1	1
diabetes mellitus	1	
HDL cholesterol <35 mg/dl	1	
HDL cholesterol >60 mg/dl	-1	
	Total:	2

Is patient at risk for complications of current conditions? ☒ Yes ☐ No
Specify: __Morbidity + mortality 2° acute asthma exacerb.__

Preventive Measures for Adults
H = has been done   R = patient refuses   X = not applicable   Date

Women		1999				
Pap Smear/pelvic	Annually 19+					
Mammogram	Every 1-2Y 40-49; annually 50+					
Men						
Rectal/prostate	Annually 50+					
All Patients						
Total/HDL-C	Every 5Y 19+	no data				
Home Fecal Occult Blood Test	Annually	R				
Immunizations						
Td	Every 10Y	H				
Influenza	Every fall*					
Pneumovax	Once*					

* if indicated

Quality of life issues

Needs Influenza vaccine

© 2000, American Society of Health-System Pharmacists, Inc. All rights reserved.

Assessment of General Appearance

Patient __Mike Kelley_____ Date _____

General Appearance	Observations and Comments

Level of consciousness
    alertness: alert, confused, delirious, stuporous, comatose,
    orientation: person, place, time
	Alert & oriented x3

Signs of distress respiratory distress, pain, anxiety, etc.	Occasional wheezes
Posture, motor activity, and gait *Describe*	Normal posture & gait
Dress, grooming, and personal hygiene *Describe*	Appropriate

Affect
    normal, inappropriate
    Describe
	Anxious about job situation and finances

Speech
    normal, impaired
    Describe
	Normal

Skin
    color: normal, blue, brown, red, pallor
    texture: normal, coarse, dry, oily
    turgor: good, poor
    edema
    lesions: color, type, configuration, anatomic distribution, consistency
	Normal - no abnormalities

Pharmacist's Patient Medical History Form

I. Patient Information

Name: __Marie Cowling__

Address: __220 East Sycamore   Sun City, AZ 21000__

Home Phone: __888-8888__   Office Phone: __N/A__

Date of Birth: __7-12-33__   Last year of education completed: __high school – 12th grade__

Patient lives with __Alone – recently widowed; new to area__

Caregiver (if applicable): __N/A__

Caregiver Phone: __N/A__

Employer: __Retired Receptionist__   Job Title: __–__

Name of Health Insurer: __MEDICARE__

Health Ins. Card #: __00-000-0000__   Social Security #: __444-44-4444__

Primary Care Physician's Name: __Dr. Dobson__   Phone: __630-218-4298 MD__

Specialist Physician's Name: __N/A__   Phone: _____

Other Health Care Practitioner: __N/A__   Phone: _____

II. Medical History

Are you allergic to any prescription drugs or over-the-counter medications? _____
☒ Yes   ☐ No   If yes, please list the medications and type of allergic reaction experienced:

__Seasonal Allergies – ragweed, pollen; Erythromycin – vomits__

Are there any medications that you are not allergic to but cannot tolerate? _____
☐ Yes   ☒ No   If yes, please list the medications and the reaction experienced:

_____

Do you use tobacco?
☐ Yes   ☒ No   If yes, what type? _____   How often? _____

Do you drink alcohol?
☒ Yes   ☐ No   If yes, what type? __Brandy__   How often? __1/wk for sleep__

Name: __Marie Cowling__

Please put a check (✔) next to those items listed below that apply to you:

HEART PROBLEMS	✔	URINARY/REPRODUCTIVE	✔
Chest pain (angina)		Urinary or bladder infection	
Past heart attack		Prostate problems	
Heart failure		Hysterectomy 20 yrs ago	✓
Irregular heartbeat		Chronic yeast infections	
Heart by-pass surgery		Kidney disease	
Rheumatic fever		Dialysis	
Other:		Other: incontinence c̄ sneezing	✓
EYES, EARS, NOSE & THROAT	✔	**MUSCLES AND BONES**	✔
Poor vision	✓	Arthritis	✓
Poor hearing	✓	Gout	
Glaucoma		Back problems	
Sinus problems		Amputation	
Balance disorder		Joint replacement	
Other:		Other:	
GASTROINTESTINAL	✔	**NEUROLOGICAL**	✔
Heartburn		Headaches	
Ulcer		Seizures or epilepsy	
Constipation		Parkinson's disease	
Diverticulitis		Dizziness	
Liver disease		Past stroke	
Gallbladder problems		Fainting	
Pancreatitis		Depression	
Other:		Anxiety	
		Other:	
DO YOU HAVE:	✔	**LUNG PROBLEMS**	✔
High blood pressure		Asthma All of life	✓
Low blood pressure		Emphysema	
High cholesterol		Bronchitis	
Diabetes		Other: Frequent colds	
Cancer			
Anemia			
Bleeding disorder		**DO YOU HAVE OR USE …?**	✔
Hay fever		Glasses	✓
Sleeping problems		Hearing aid	
Other:		Other:	
DO YOU HAVE A FAMILY HISTORY OF:			
High blood pressure		Asthma	
Heart disease	✓	Other: Breast Cancer	✓
Diabetes			

Name: Marie Cowling

III. CURRENT PRESCRIPTION MEDICATIONS (INCLUDING ONES RECEIVED AT OTHER PHARMACIES)

Name of prescription medicine and strength (i.e., milligrams, grams, and units)	How much do you take each time?	How many times a day do you take the medicine?	Medical problem being treated	When did you start taking this medicine?	Has the medicine helped you? Yes/No	Name of doctor or specialist who prescribed the medicine
Example: Diabeta, 2.5 mg	1	2	Diabetes	1992	Yes	Dr. Harold Smith
Maxair MDI	2 puffs	3	Asthma	? years	?	Dobson

IV. CURRENT NONPRESCRIPTION MEDICATIONS

Ex: ANTACIDS, ANTI-DIARRHEALS, ALLERGY MEDICINES, ANTI-NAUSEA, DIET PILLS, EAR OR EYE MEDICATIONS, LAXATIVES, PAIN RELIEVERS, VITAMINS, ETC.

Name of medicine Example: Tylenol	How often do you take it? (daily, once a week, etc.)	Name of medicine	How often do you take it?
Motrin 200 mg	2x/day (take 2 tabs)		
One-a-Day w/ calcium	1/day		

I certify this information is accurate and complete to the best of my knowledge. _Marie Cowling_ _7/8/99_
                                                                    signature   date

© 2000, American Society of Health-System Pharmacists, Inc. All rights reserved.

Pharmacist's Patient Database Form

Original Date:_____
Date updated:_____
Date updated:_____
Date updated:_____

Demographic and Administrative Information

Name:	Social Security #:
Address:	
Health Care Provider's Name	Health Care Provider's Phone
Work Phone: Home Phone:	Date of Birth:
Race:	Gender:
Religion:	Occupation:
Health Insurer:	Subscriber #:
Primary Card Holder:	Drug Benefit: ❑ yes ❑ no copay: $_____

Current Symptoms

Past Medical History	Acute and Current Medical Problems
	1.
	2.
	3.
	4.
	5.
	6.
	7.
	8.

Family/Social/Economic History	Personal Limitations

Cost of medications per month $_____

Allergies/Intolerances	Social Drug Use
❑ No known drug allergies	Alcohol
Medication Reaction	Caffeine
	Tobacco
	Pregnancy/Breastfeeding Status
	❑ Pregnant (due _____) ❑ Breastfeeding

Diet	Routine Exercise/Recreation	Daily Activities/Timing
❑ Low salt		
❑ Low fat		
❑ Diabetic		
Timing of meals:		

© 2000, American Society of Health-System Pharmacists, Inc. All rights reserved.

Patient Name: _____

Physical Assessment/Laboratory Data—Initial/Follow-up					
Date					
Height					
Weight					
Temp					
BP					
Pulse					
Respirations					
Peak Flow					
FBG					
R. Glucose					
HbA$_{1c}$					
T. Chol.					
LDL					
HDL					
TG					
INR					
BUN					
Cr					
ALT					
AST					
Alk Phos					

Drug Serum Concentrations

Date					

Notes:

© 2000, American Society of Health-System Pharmacists, Inc. All rights reserved.

Patient Name: _____

Current Prescription Medication Regimen

Name/Dose/Strength/Route	Schedule/Frequency of Use	Indication	Start Date (and Stop Date If Applicable)	Prescriber	Adherence Issues/Efficacy

Current Nonprescription Medication Regimen (OTC, herbal, homeopathic, nutritional, etc.)

Name/Dose/Strength/Route	Schedule/Frequency of Use	Indication	Start Date (and Stop Date If Applicable)	Prescriber	Adherence Issues/Efficacy

©2000, American Society of Health-System Pharmacists, Inc. All rights reserved.

Patient Name: _____

Risk Assessment/Preventive Measures/Quality of Life

Cardiovascular Risk Assessment		
male >45 years old	1	
female >55 years old or female <55 with history of ovarectomy not taking estrogen replacement	1	
Definite MI or sudden death before age 55 year in father or male first-degree relative or before 65 year in mother or female first-degree relative	1	
current cigarette smoking	1	
hypertension	1	
diabetes mellitus	1	
HDL cholesterol <35 mg/dl	1	
HDL cholesterol >60 mg/dl	-1	
	Total:	

Is patient at risk for complications of current conditions? ❑ Yes ❑ No
Specify:

Preventive Measures for Adults
H = has been done   R = patient refuses   X = not applicable   Date

Women							
Pap Smear/pelvic	Annually 19+						
Mammogram	Every 1-2Y 40-49; annually 50+						
Men							
Rectal/prostate	Annually 50+						
All Patients							
Total/HDL-C	Every 5Y 19+						
Home Fecal Occult Blood Test	Annually						
Immunizations							
Td	Every 10Y						
Influenza	Every fall*						
Pneumovax	Once*						

* if indicated

Quality of life issues

© 2000, American Society of Health-System Pharmacists, Inc. All rights reserved.

Assessment of General Appearance

Patient _____ Date _____

General Appearance	Observations and Comments

Level of consciousness
    alertness: alert, confused,
    delirious, stuporous, comatose,
    orientation: person, place, time	

Signs of distress respiratory distress, pain, anxiety, etc.	
Posture, motor activity, and gait *Describe*	
Dress, grooming, and personal hygiene *Describe*	

Affect
    normal, inappropriate
    Describe	

Speech
    normal, impaired
    Describe	

Skin
    color: normal, blue, brown, red, pallor
    texture: normal, coarse, dry, oily
    turgor: good, poor
    edema
    lesions: color, type, configuration, anatomic
       distribution, consistency	

Pharmacist's Patient Database Form

Original Date: **7/8/99**
Date updated: _____
Date updated: _____
Date updated: _____

Demographic and Administrative Information

Name: Marie Cowling
Social Security #: 444-44-4444
Address: 220 East Sycamore, Sun City, AZ
Health Care Provider's Name: Dr. Dobson
Health Care Provider's Phone: 630-218-4298
Work Phone: N/A
Home Phone:
Date of Birth: 7-12-33
Race: White
Gender: Female
Religion: N/A
Occupation: Retired
Health Insurer: MediCare
Subscriber #: 00-000-0000
Primary Card Holder: Marie
Drug Benefit: ☒ yes ☐ no copay: $10.00

Current Symptoms

Breathing difficulties

Past Medical History

- hysterectomy ~20 yrs ago
- Breathing problems – periodic through all of adult life
- Frequent colds

Acute and Current Medical Problems

1. Breathing Difficulties
2. Allergies
3. Arthritis
4.
5.
6.
7.
8.

Family/Social/Economic History

- recently widowed
- retired
- 2 children – adult; living in Minneapolis
- Moved to Sun City – 6 wks ago

Cost of medications per month $20.00

Personal Limitations

None

Allergies/Intolerances

☒ No known drug allergies

Medication	Reaction
Erythromycin	GI intolerance

Social Drug Use

- Alcohol: occasional
- Caffeine: None
- Tobacco: None

Pregnancy/Breastfeeding Status

☐ Pregnant (due _____) ☐ Breastfeeding

Diet

☐ Low salt
☐ Low fat
☐ Diabetic
Timing of meals:

Routine Exercise/Recreation

walks 2 miles daily

Daily Activities/Timing

Patient Name: **Marie Cowling**

Physical Assessment/Laboratory Data—Initial/Follow-up

Date	7/8/99				
Height					
Weight					
Temp					
BP					
Pulse					
Respirations					
Peak Flow					
FBG					
R. Glucose					
HbA_{1c}					
T. Chol.					
LDL					
HDL					
TG					
INR					
BUN					
Cr					
ALT					
AST					
Alk Phos					
WBC	7.2				
Diff	85s 2b 13L				
Pulse Ox	95%				

Drug Serum Concentrations

Date					

Notes:

© 2000, American Society of Health-System Pharmacists, Inc. All rights reserved.

Patient Name: Marie Cowling

Current Prescription Medication Regimen

Name/Dose/Strength/Route	Schedule/Frequency of Use	Indication	Start Date (and Stop Date If Applicable)	Prescriber	Adherence Issues/Efficacy
Maxair MDI	2 puffs Q 8° pm	Asthma	years	Dobson	↑ frequency of use – 2 refill in 6 wks

Current Nonprescription Medication Regimen (OTC, herbal, homeopathic, nutritional, etc.)

Name/Dose/Strength/Route	Schedule/Frequency of Use	Indication	Start Date (and Stop Date If Applicable)	Prescriber	Adherence Issues/Efficacy
ibuprofen 200 mg	2 tabs BID	Arthritis	years	—	
One-A-Day with calcium	One/day	Supplement	years	—	

©2000, American Society of Health-System Pharmacists, Inc. All rights reserved.

Patient Name: Marie Cowling

Risk Assessment/Preventive Measures/Quality of Life

Cardiovascular Risk Assessment		
male >45 years old	1	
female >55 years old or female <55 with history of ovarectomy not taking estrogen replacement	1	1
Definite MI or sudden death before age 55 year in father or male first-degree relative or before 65 year in mother or female first-degree relative	1	
current cigarette smoking	1	
hypertension	1	
diabetes mellitus	1	
HDL cholesterol <35 mg/dl	1	?
HDL cholesterol >60 mg/dl	-1	?
	Total:	

Is patient at risk for complications of current conditions? ☒ Yes ☐ No
Specify: Acute Exacerbation → Morbidity / Mortality

Preventive Measures for Adults H = has been done R = patient refuses X = not applicable		Date				
Women		2/99				
Pap Smear/pelvic	Annually 19+	X				
Mammogram	Every 1-2Y 40-49; annually 50+	H				
Men						
Rectal/prostate	Annually 50+					
All Patients						
Total/HDL-C	Every 5Y 19+	?				
Home Fecal Occult Blood Test	Annually					
Immunizations						
Td	Every 10Y	H				
Influenza	Every fall*	H				
Pneumovax	Once*	H				

* if indicated

Quality of life issues

Patient alone and fearful - breathing difficulties
Controlling her life - moved to Sun City upon suggestion of
MD → to improve breathing + arthritis

© 2000, American Society of Health-System Pharmacists, Inc. All rights reserved.

Assessment of General Appearance

Patient **Marie Cowling** Date _____

General Appearance	Observations and Comments

Level of consciousness
    alertness: alert, confused, delirious, stuporous, comatose,
    orientation: person, place, time
	Alert & oriented x3

Signs of distress respiratory distress, pain, anxiety, etc.	None
Posture, motor activity, and gait *Describe*	Normal posture & gait
Dress, grooming, and personal hygiene *Describe*	Appropriate

Affect
    normal, inappropriate
    Describe
	Normal - somewhat sad - all alone

Speech
    normal, impaired
    Describe
	Normal

Skin
    color: normal, blue, brown, red, pallor
    texture: normal, coarse, dry, oily
    turgor: good, poor
    edema
    lesions: color, type, configuration, anatomic distribution, consistency
	Normal
	No abnormalities

Appendix G 89

Pharmacist's Patient Medical History Form

I. Patient Information

Name: __Mary Franklin__
Address: __121 College Dorm Way   Cowtown, USA 19776__
Home Phone: __888-7777__   Office Phone: _____
Date of Birth: __3-4-80__   Last year of education completed: __freshman year coll. - curr.__
Patient lives with __Roommate__
Caregiver (if applicable): __N/A__
Caregiver Phone: __N/A__
Employer: __N/A student__   Job Title: _____
Name of Health Insurer: __Student Health__
Health Ins. Card #: __1213489__   Social Security #: __133-33-0333__
Primary Care Physician's Name: __Dr. Faraway__   Phone: __?__
Specialist Physician's Name: __N/A__   Phone: _____
Other Health Care Practitioner: __N/A__   Phone: _____

II. Medical History

Are you allergic to any prescription drugs or over-the-counter medications? _____
❏ Yes   ☒ No   If yes, please list the medications and type of allergic reaction experienced:

_____

Are there any medications that you are not allergic to but cannot tolerate? _____
❏ Yes   ☒ No   If yes, please list the medications and the reaction experienced:

_____

Do you use tobacco?
❏ Yes   ☒ No   If yes, what type? _____   How often? _____

Do you drink alcohol?
☒ Yes   ❏ No   If yes, what type? __Beer__   How often? __2 nights/week__

Name: **Mary Franklin**

Please put a check (✔) next to those items listed below that apply to you:

HEART PROBLEMS	✔	URINARY/REPRODUCTIVE	✔
Chest pain (angina)		Urinary or bladder infection	
Past heart attack		Prostate problems	
Heart failure		Hysterectomy	
Irregular heartbeat		Chronic yeast infections	
Heart by-pass surgery		Kidney disease	
Rheumatic fever		Dialysis	
Other:		Other:	
EYES, EARS, NOSE & THROAT	✔	**MUSCLES AND BONES**	✔
Poor vision Contacts	✓	Arthritis	
Poor hearing		Gout	
Glaucoma		Back problems	
Sinus problems		Amputation	
Balance disorder		Joint replacement	
Other:		Other:	
GASTROINTESTINAL	✔	**NEUROLOGICAL**	✔
Heartburn		Headaches	
Ulcer		Seizures or epilepsy	
Constipation		Parkinson's disease	
Diverticulitis		Dizziness	
Liver disease		Past stroke	
Gallbladder problems		Fainting	
Pancreatitis		Depression	
Other:		Anxiety	
		Other:	
DO YOU HAVE:	✔	**LUNG PROBLEMS**	✔
High blood pressure		Asthma	✓
Low blood pressure		Emphysema	
High cholesterol		Bronchitis	
Diabetes		Other:	
Cancer			
Anemia			
Bleeding disorder		**DO YOU HAVE OR USE …?**	✔
Hay fever		Glasses	
Sleeping problems		Hearing aid	
Other:		Other:	
DO YOU HAVE A FAMILY HISTORY OF:			
High blood pressure		Asthma	
Heart disease	✓	Other:	
Diabetes			

Name: __Mary Franklin__

III. Current Prescription Medications (Including Ones Received at Other Pharmacies)

Name of prescription medicine and strength (i.e., milligrams, grams, and units)	How much do you take each time?	How many times a day do you take the medicine?	Medical problem being treated	When did you start taking this medicine?	Has the medicine helped you? Yes/No	Name of doctor or specialist who prescribed the medicine
Example: Diabeta, 2.5 mg	1	2	Diabetes	1992	Yes	Dr. Harold Smith
Proventil inhaler	2-3 puffs	several	asthma	years	yes	Dr. Faraway

IV. Current Nonprescription Medications

Ex: antacids, anti-diarrheals, allergy medicines, anti-nausea, diet pills, ear or eye medications, laxatives, pain relievers, vitamins, etc.

Name of medicine Example: Tylenol	How often do you take it? (daily, once a week, etc.)	Name of medicine	How often do you take it?
Tylenol	2 capsules - 2x/week		
ibuprofen 200 mg	2 tablets - once a month		

I certify this information is accurate and complete to the best of my knowledge. __Mary Franklin__ __9/20/99__
                                                                                   signature   date

© 2000, American Society of Health-System Pharmacists, Inc. All rights reserved.

Pharmacist's Patient Database Form

Original Date: 9/20/99
Date updated: _____
Date updated: _____
Date updated: _____

Demographic and Administrative Information

Name: Mary Franklin	Social Security #: 133-33-0333
Address: 121 College Dorm Way Cowtown, USA 19776	
Health Care Provider's Name: Dr. Faraway	Health Care Provider's Phone: can't remember
Work Phone: Home Phone: 888-7777	Date of Birth: 3/4/80
Race: White	Gender: F
Religion: ∅	Occupation:
Health Insurer: Student Health	Subscriber #: 1213489
Primary Card Holder: Mary Franklin	Drug Benefit: ☒ yes ☐ no copay: $ 15

Current Symptoms

↑'d need for albuterol inhaler

Past Medical History	Acute and Current Medical Problems
Asthma since childhood	1.
	2.
	3.
	4.
	5.
	6.
	7.
	8.

Family/Social/Economic History	Personal Limitations
College Freshman	∅

Cost of medications per month $ _____

Allergies/Intolerances	Social Drug Use	
☒ No known drug allergies	Alcohol	beer 2 nights/week - several
Medication Reaction	Caffeine	Pepsi - 3/day
	Tobacco	
	Pregnancy/Breastfeeding Status	
	☐ Pregnant (due _____) ☐ Breastfeeding	

Diet	Routine Exercise/Recreation	Daily Activities/Timing
☐ Low salt		Classes
☐ Low fat		Aerobics - 3x/week -
☐ Diabetic		needs inhaler
Timing of meals:		

Patient Name: Mary Franklin

Physical Assessment/Laboratory Data—Initial/Follow-up

Date	9/20/99	10/31/99			
Height	5'4"	5'4"			
Weight	115 lbs	115 lbs			
Temp					
BP					
Pulse					
Respirations	16	14			
Peak Flow					
FBG					
R. Glucose					
HbA_{1c}					
T. Chol.					
LDL					
HDL					
TG					
INR					
BUN					
Cr					
ALT					
AST					
Alk Phos					

Drug Serum Concentrations

Date					

Notes: 9/20 referred to local MD (names given) for asthma eval., ↑ use of albuterol

Patient Name: Mary Franklin

Current Prescription Medication Regimen

Name/Dose/Strength/Route	Schedule/Frequency of Use	Indication	Start Date (and Stop Date If Applicable)	Prescriber	Adherence Issues/Efficacy
Proventil MDI	2-3 puffs 5-6x/day	wheezing	years	Dr. Faraway	*↑ use, no action plan

Current Nonprescription Medication Regimen (OTC, herbal, homeopathic, nutritional, etc.)

Name/Dose/Strength/Route	Schedule/Frequency of Use	Indication	Start Date (and Stop Date If Applicable)	Prescriber	Adherence Issues/Efficacy
Tylenol	2 tabs prn	HA	years	—	
Ibuprofen 200 mg	2 tabs prn	Cramps	years	—	

©2000, American Society of Health-System Pharmacists, Inc. All rights reserved.

Patient Name: Mary Franklin

Risk Assessment/Preventive Measures/Quality of Life

Cardiovascular Risk Assessment		
male >45 years old	1	
female >55 years old or female <55 with history of ovarectomy not taking estrogen replacement	1	
Definite MI or sudden death before age 55 year in father or male first-degree relative or before 65 year in mother or female first-degree relative	1	
current cigarette smoking	1	
hypertension	1	
diabetes mellitus	1	
HDL cholesterol <35 mg/dl	1	
HDL cholesterol >60 mg/dl	-1	-1
	Total:	-1

Is patient at risk for complications of current conditions? ☑ Yes ☐ No
Specify: Uncontrolled asthma exacerbation

Preventive Measures for Adults H = has been done R = patient refuses X = not applicable		Date				
Women		8/99				
Pap Smear/pelvic	Annually 19+	H				
Mammogram	Every 1-2Y 40-49; annually 50+					
Men						
Rectal/prostate	Annually 50+					
All Patients						
Total/HDL-C	Every 5Y 19+	H				
Home Fecal Occult Blood Test	Annually					
Immunizations						
Td	Every 10Y	H				
Influenza	Every fall*	H				
Pneumovax	Once*					

* if indicated

Quality of life issues

Pt c̄ ↑ need for Beta-adrenergic agonist; sent for eval –
? need for inhaled steroid. – will f/u in 1 wk.

© 2000, American Society of Health-System Pharmacists, Inc. All rights reserved.

Assessment of General Appearance

Patient **Mary Franklin**   Date **9/20/99**

General Appearance	Observations and Comments
Level of consciousness 　alertness: alert, confused, 　delirious, stuporous, comatose, 　orientation: person, place, time	Alert & oriented x3
Signs of distress 　respiratory distress, pain, anxiety, etc.	None
Posture, motor activity, and gait 　*Describe*	Normal
Dress, grooming, and personal hygiene 　*Describe*	Appropriate
Affect 　normal, inappropriate 　*Describe*	Initially angry, scared due to no support system
Speech 　normal, impaired 　*Describe*	Normal
Skin 　color: normal, blue, brown, red, pallor 　texture: normal, coarse, dry, oily 　turgor: good, poor 　edema 　lesions: color, type, configuration, anatomic 　　distribution, consistency	Normal

Part II

Developing an Ambulatory Pharmacist's Care Plan for Patients with Asthma

Assessing Current Medication Therapy and Creating a Therapy Problem List

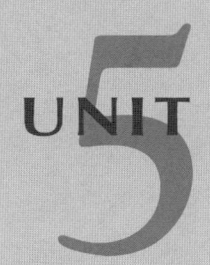

UNIT 5

Unit Objectives	100
Unit Organization	100
Common Therapy Problems of Ambulatory Care Patients with Asthma	100
Example Case 1	101
Example Case 2	103
Case Study: Determining the Presence of Therapy Problems	104
Case Study: Prioritizing Problems	104
Practice Example: Constructing the Therapy Problem List	105
Summary	106
References	106
Self-Study Questions	107
Self-Study Answers	108
Appendixes	109

Unit 8 of the *Ambulatory Care Clinical Skills Program: Core Module* provided a standardized approach to the assessment of a patient's medications and the creation of a therapy problem list. The ambulatory care pharmacist interested in managing patients with asthma will need to follow this basic approach, modifying it to meet the unique needs of patients with asthma. Because asthma is a chronic illness that is episodic in nature, patient drug therapy problems will most likely vary from visit to visit. In this unit, we will discuss specific problems that may require a pharmacist to alter the therapy of ambulatory care patients with asthma.

Unit Objectives

After you successfully complete this unit, you will be able to:
- describe types of problems commonly present in the unreviewed therapy of ambulatory care patients with asthma;
- determine the presence of any of the following medication or related therapy problems in the current therapy of ambulatory care patients with asthma:
  - medication used with no medical indication;
  - medical condition for which there is no medication prescribed;
  - medication prescribed inappropriately for particular medical condition;
  - incomplete immunization status;
  - anything inappropriate in the current medication therapy regimen (dose, dosage form, schedule, duration, route of administration, or method of administration);
  - presence of therapeutic duplication;
  - prescription of medication to which the patient is allergic;
  - presence or potential for adverse drug events;
  - presence or potential for clinically significant drug-drug, drug-disease, drug-nutrient, or drug–laboratory test interactions;
  - interference with medical therapy by social or cultural drug use or use of alternative therapies (e.g., herbal or homeopathic therapies);
  - problems arising from financial impact of medication therapy on the patient;
  - patient lack of understanding of medication therapy;
  - patient not adhering to medication regimen;
  - patient at risk for complications associated with asthma or another disease;
  - patient at risk because of patient-specific characteristics (e.g., age or living/working environment); or
  - therapy is adversely impacting patient's quality of life;
- explain factors that are unique to ambulatory care patients with asthma to be considered when prioritizing their medication or related problems;
- explain special concerns in the prioritization of medication and related health care problems for ambulatory care patients with asthma; and
- construct a therapy problem list for ambulatory care patients with asthma.

Unit Organization

This unit will begin with a discussion of common therapy problems unique to ambulatory care patients with asthma. Next, a determination of therapy-related problems and prioritization of these problems will be addressed. Finally, the actual construction of a therapy problem list will be covered.

Common Therapy Problems of Ambulatory Care Patients with Asthma

Adherence to a prescribed therapy is one of the most common problems with any type of drug therapy. Nonadherence is especially problematic in asthma. The chronic nature of the disease requires that patients with persistent asthma take an anti-inflammatory medication to help control and prevent asthma exacerbations. Successful asthma management requires the adherence of a patient to a treatment regimen. Statistics have shown, however, that <40% of patients adhere to a given regimen.[1] Poor adherence to a prescribed treatment regimen is associated with increased mortality due to asthma.[2] Adherence to a prescribed regimen can be affected by many factors:
- fear of addiction to medications;
- fear that the medication won't work;
- fear of long-term side effects;
- fear of being different;
- inability to administer medications (because

of lack of privacy, no time, or fears about job security);
- misconceptions about medications;
- no plan of therapy;
- complexity of the regimen;
- adverse effects; or
- financial concerns.

When patients are not feeling the effects of their disease, adherence to a medication regimen can be particularly difficult. It is hard to maintain adherence when one doesn't feel sick and therefore may not see the benefit of taking a medication. Patients need to be educated about the chronic nature of their disease and the need for prophylactic maintenance therapy when prescribed. Informing patients about the potential mortality associated with uncontrolled asthma should help them understand the need to adhere to a prescribed therapy.

In addition, many patients fear becoming addicted to their medications. Asthma patients often fear addiction to steroids. They are not always aware of the differences between corticosteroids and anabolic steroids. Pharmacists need to be mindful of this fact and be sure that the patient and/or caregivers understand the differences between these drugs.

As mentioned in the first unit of this module, when patients are included in the decisions about therapy goals, they will be more likely to adhere to a prescribed therapy. The long-term effects of beta$_2$-adrenergic agonists and corticosteroids have received a lot of attention in both the media and scientific literature over the past several years. Pharmacists should be able to discuss this risk-benefit information with the patient in simple language to alleviate fears about the side effects.

Adherence can also be affected by the desire of a patient to not stand out from others because of the need to take a medication. This desire is especially relevant in the pediatric and adolescent populations, but it can also be found in the adult population. In some educational and work settings, it may be difficult for a person to administer their inhaled medication in a private setting, making the patient less likely to take medication on a regular basis. Patient knowledge about medications is an important aspect of care and can affect adherence. Patients who do not have an understanding of the intent of each medication (control vs. relief) and how it works to treat asthma will be less adherent than those who understand why each medication is prescribed.

Patients with asthma should have a treatment plan to follow that they develop with their physician. Patients who believe they can have a positive impact on their disease by adhering to a treatment plan will be more likely to follow a prescribed regimen.[1] As a pharmacist, you should help the patient adhere to this plan and make sure that the patient understands and is able to carry out the steps outlined in the treatment plan.

Duplication of medications can be a significant issue for patients with asthma. Duplicate short-acting beta$_2$-adrenergic agonists or corticosteroids may be noted during a patient medication history. Patients may not recognize that two albuterol inhalers may indeed be the same medication with a different brand name. Patients may quite often continue taking a medication after it has been discontinued when instructions are unclear. Patients who use nebulizers sometimes employ albuterol as the diluent for other medications and do not recognize it as a medication and may be using an oral inhaler as well. Duplication of therapy can lead to toxicity, increased expense, and decreased adherence.

Another important consideration arises from therapeutic interchange. Many prescription plans approve only one or two inhaled corticosteroids on the formulary. This creates a situation where therapeutic interchange may take place. Therapeutic interchange of a nonpreferred (nonformulary) drug for a preferred (formulary) drug is common in many settings today, especially in the managed care arena. As a pharmacist you should make sure that, when an interchange occurs, the correct number of puffs/day have been prescribed. Many times, the interchange takes place without consideration for ensuring an equivalent dose of the preferred agent. The equivalency issue is most important for patients that are stabilized on one drug and then switched to another agent within the same class. Under- or overdosing can create problems for a patient. **Table 1** compares daily dosages for inhaled corticosteroids.

Example Case 1

Jake Conser is a 10-year-old child with six emergency room visits in the past 12 months due to asthma exacerbations. He has been maintained on cromolyn and as-needed albuterol for the past year. With the most recent trip to the emergency room,

Table 1. Estimated Comparative Daily Dosages for Inhaled Corticosteroids

Adults

Drug	Low Dose	Medium Dose	High Dose
Beclomethasone dipropionate 42 μg/puff 84 μg/puff	168–504 μg (4–12 puffs—42 μg) (2–6 puffs—84 μg)	504–840 μg (12–20 puffs—42 μg) (6–10 puffs—84 μg)	>840 μg (>20 puffs—42 μg) (>10 puffs—84 μg)
Budesonide DPI: 200 μg/dose	200–400 μg (1–2 inhalations)	400–600 μg (2–3 inhalations)	>600 μg (>3 inhalations)
Flunisolide 250 μg/puff	500–1000 μg (2–4 puffs)	1000–2000 μg (4–8 puffs)	>2000 μg (>8 puffs)
Fluticasone MDI: 44, 110, 220 μg/puff	88–264 μg (2–6 puffs—44 μg) OR (2 puffs—110 μg)	264–660 μg (2–6 puffs—110 μg)	>660 μg (>6 puffs—110 μg) OR (>3 puffs—220 μg)
DPI: 50, 100, 250 μg/dose	(2–6 inhalations—50 μg)	(3–6 inhalations—100 μg)	(>6 inhalations—100 μg) OR (>2 inhalations—250 μg)
Triamcinolone acetonide 100 μg/puff	400–1000 μg (4–10 puffs)	1000–2000 μg (10–20 puffs)	>2000 μg (>20 puffs)

Children

Drug	Low Dose	Medium Dose	High Dose
Beclomethasone dipropionate 42 μg/puff 84 μg/puff	84–336 μg (2–8 puffs—42 μg) (1–4 puffs—84 μg)	336–672 μg (8–16 puffs—42 μg) (4–8 puffs—84 μg)	>672 μg (>16 puffs—42 μg) (>8 puffs—84 μg)
Budesonide DPI: 200 μg/dose	100–200 μg	200–400 μg (1–2 inhalations—200 μg)	>400 μg (>2 inhalations — 200 μg)
Flunisolide 250 μg/puff	500–750 μg (2–3 puffs)	1000–1250 μg (4–5 puffs)	>1250 μg (>5 puffs)
Fluticasone MDI: 44, 110, 220 μg/puff	88–176 μg (2–4 puffs—44 μg)	176–440 μg (4–10 puffs—44 μg) OR (2–4 puffs—110 μg)	>440 μg (>4 puffs—110 μg) OR (>2 puffs—220 μg)
DPI: 50, 100, 250 μg/dose	(2–4 inhalations—50 μg)	(2–4 inhalations—100 μg)	(>4 inhalations—100 μg) OR (>2 inhalations—250 μg)
Triamcinolone acetonide 100 μg/puff	400–800 μg (4–8 puffs)	800–1200 μg (8–12 puffs)	>1200 μg (>12 puffs)

Source: reprinted with permission from reference 4.

> **Notes:**
> - The most important determinant of appropriate dosing is the clinician's judgment of the patient's response to therapy. The clinician must monitor the patient's response on several clinical parameters and adjust the dose accordingly. The stepwise approach to therapy emphasizes that once control of asthma is achieved, the dose of medication should be carefully titrated to the minimum dose required to maintain control, thus reducing the potential for adverse effects.
> - See reference 4 for an explanation of the rationale used for the comparative dosages. The reference point for the range in the dosages for children is data on the safety of inhaled corticosteroids in children, which, in general, suggest that the dose ranges are equivalent to beclomethasone dipropionate 200–400 μg/day (low dose), 400–800 μg/day (medium dose), and >800 μg/day (high dose).
> - Some dosages may be outside package labeling.
> - Metered-dose inhaler (MDI) dosages are expressed as the actuater dose (the amount of drug leaving the actuater and delivered to the patient), which is the labeling required in the United States. This is different from the dosage expressed as the valve dose (the amount of drug leaving the valve, all of which is not available to the patient), which is used in many European countries and in some of the scientific literature. Dry powder inhaler (DPI) doses are expressed as the amount of drug in the inhaler following activation.

his physician decided to begin flunisolide and discontinue the cromolyn. Mrs. Conser brings the prescription to the pharmacy to be filled.

Mrs. Conser:
"Hi Sue! I'm here to get a new medicine for Jake. His asthma seems to be getting worse and the doctor wants to start him on a steroid. I'm not too sure about this. I've heard all about those kids that abuse these steroids so that they can be better athletes. I'm worried about what this will do to Jake. I also heard something the other night on the news about the steroids stopping bone growth. This doesn't sounds like something I want Jake to have to take."

Pharmacist:
"I know all of the information you hear can be confusing. Why don't we step over here and talk about the differences between the steroids you hear about people abusing and this one. We can also talk about the effects on bone growth. In Jake's case, the risk of him having a problem from his asthma is much greater than the side effects from the drugs."

Situations such as Jake's are not uncommon. They can also arise in the elderly population because of concerns regarding the long-term effects of corticosteroids on glaucoma. Pharmacists need to be equipped to handle these discussions and need to keep up-to-date with the latest information about asthma medications.

Example Case 2

Nicole is a 4-year-old child with a diagnosis of asthma. Her mother administers her medications with a nebulizer. Until now, she has been receiving cromolyn and albuterol via nebulization. Her mother was instructed to use the cromolyn (rather than saline) to dilute the albuterol. At her last visit, the cromolyn was discontinued and she was placed on an inhaled corticosteroid. (This was noted in the patient's progress note.) When the pharmacist reviewed her medication history, the mother indicated she was still using the cromolyn to dilute Nicole's albuterol. No one had instructed her to do things differently. The continued use of cromolyn not only exposed Nicole to an extra medication, but also increased the overall expense of Nicole's care.

Overuse of beta$_2$-adrenergic agonists can be a problem for many patients and may be more common among patients who are busy or do not like to seek medical attention. This overuse is a sign of asthma that is not adequately controlled. Patients who do not recognize the extent of their worsening symptoms may also overuse their beta$_2$-adrenergic agonists. In any patient, the beta$_2$-adrenergic agonists may be overused as a means to gain control of an acute exacerbation without seeking medical attention. Overreliance on beta$_2$-adrenergic agonists may delay needed medical care, placing the patient in danger. The majority of deaths from asthma occur outside medical facilities, most likely because failure to recognize the severity of symptoms led to a delay in seeking medical help.[3] Exacerbations may be due to nonadherence, worsening disease, concurrent disease states, inappropriate medication regimens (need for an anti-inflammatory agent), or exposure to a trigger. Patients who require more than one canister of a short-acting beta$_2$-adrenergic agonist a month or one every 2 months when it is used in conjunction with a long-acting beta$_2$-adrenergic agonists should be reassessed.[4] An ambulatory care pharmacist who identifies overuse of beta$_2$-adrenergic agonists should take the opportunity both to educate the patient and notify the patient's physician. A change in therapy may be necessary.

Case Study: Determining the Presence of Therapy Problems

In this section, we will use a case study to learn how to determine the presence of therapy problems in a patient with asthma. The Ambulatory Therapy Assessment Worksheet (ATAW) introduced in unit 8 of the *Core Module* will be helpful in this process, you may want to review this unit before going any further. The ATAW provides a systematic approach to the review of a patient's medication regimen and therapy plan.

We will return to the case of Jeremy Morgan for this exercise. You will need to use the Pharmacist's Patient Medical History Form and Pharmacist's Patient Database Form found in **Appendix A** for this exercise. Follow along as we review the completed ATAW in Appendix A.

Correlation between drug therapy and medical problems:
- A problem exists: Echinacea has been used for >1 year; immunostimulating effects diminish with prolonged use.

Appropriate therapy:
- A problem exists: therapy not meeting desired outcomes; overuse of albuterol.

Drug regimen:
- A problem exists: patient taking ibuprofen, may exacerbate symptoms. Need to determine whether Jeremy's symptoms worsen when taking ibuprofen.

Therapeutic duplication:
- A problem exists: albuterol MDI and nebs.

Drug allergy or intolerance:
- No problem exists.

Adverse drug events:
- No problem exists.

Interactions: Drug-drug, drug-disease, drug-nutrient, drug-laboratory test:
- A problem exists: ibuprofen may exacerbate symptoms.

Social or recreational drug use:
- A problem exists: tobacco and alcohol experimentation.

Financial impact:
- No problem exists.

Patient knowledge of therapy:
- A problem exists: Jeremy and his mother are unsure of medications use and risk vs. benefit.

Adherence:
- A problem exists; medication refill history: corticosteroid use nonadherent; increased exacerbations.

Self-monitoring:
- A problem exists: Jeremy does not consistently perform peak-flow measurements.

Risks and quality of life impacts:
- A problem exists: adolescent downplaying need for medications and worsening symptoms, at risk for severe episode or death; needs influenza vaccine, patient quality of life is decreasing because of increased exacerbations; sleep disrupted.

Case Study: Prioritizing Problems

As you can see from Jeremy's completed ATAW, he has several problems that have been identified. The question now is to prioritize the problems so that appropriate actions can be taken. In the case of Jeremy, his failure to adhere to therapy places him at high risk for developing a severe or even fatal asthma exacerbation. This intervention is most likely the most important one for Jeremy at this time. Education about the risk of asthma and the goals of his treatment plan should help convince Jeremy to be more adherent. Jeremy's mother should be included in these discussions. Mrs. Morgan has been struggling with giving Jeremy responsibility for his medications and control of his disease. Jeremy is probably not quite ready for all of that responsibility.

Mrs. Morgan has also been hesitant to enforce

the use of inhaled corticosteroids because she is uncertain about their long-term effects. Educating both Jeremy and his mother about this class of drugs will be required. Peak flow monitoring education will need to be completed and can be done during the next visit or two. The more important factor for Jeremy at this time is to help him become adherent and to get him to avoid triggers (specifically tobacco). You need to determine whether ibuprofen is responsible for precipitating any of Jeremy's asthma exacerbations. You must also educate both Jeremy and his mother about the potential for ibuprofen to precipitate an exacerbation and provide him with alternatives for pain relief. The list of drugs that patients with asthma need to avoid is not extensive. However, about 5–20% of asthma patients are aspirin sensitive.[3] Patients who are aspirin sensitive may also be sensitive to nonsteroidal anti-inflammatory drugs (NSAIDs). Aspirin and NSAID sensitivity may be manifested as rhinorrhea, wheezing, or shortness of breath, which can be life threatening. Although this reaction is not universal among patients with asthma, it is best to have aspirin-sensitive patients avoid these agents all together. Some clinicians suggest that all patients avoid these agents. Patients with asthma should also avoid beta-adrenergic-blockers, especially nonselective beta-adrenergic-blockers. The issue of influenza vaccination is a much lower priority and can wait until a future visit. Education about proper inhaler technique and reinforcement of the therapy plan will need to be conducted with each patient-pharmacist interaction.

Prioritizing patient needs will differ, depending on the patient, the patient's history and immediate needs, the patient's current state of health, the goals of therapy, financial concerns, and the patient's willingness to adhere to therapy. Prioritizing patient needs will need to be performed at each visit, as patients' lives will be constantly changing. Financial issues will be a higher priority for patients without insurance than for patients with insurance. Patients with changing environmental or seasonal exacerbations will also need to have their problems reprioritized with each encounter. The patient's needs and goals of therapy should always be given top priority when ranking and determining problem priorities. Patients who see multiple practitioners for control of their disease (e.g., primary physician, chiropractor, acupuncturist, nutritionist, and practitioner of other forms of alternative medicine) should be encouraged to share information with each provider so that the goals of therapy can be melded together. This way the practitioners can work in unison for the common goal of improving the patient's asthma control and quality of life. Refer to the therapy problem list (TPL) of the Ambulatory Pharmacist Care Plan (APCP) in Appendix A to see how Jeremy's problem list was recorded.

Practice Example: Constructing the Therapy Problem List

Now that we have talked about prioritizing therapy problems and practiced going through Jeremy's ATAW, you will have a chance to develop a therapy problem list (TPL) on your own. For this exercise, use the information in **Appendix B** for Mr. Kelley. You have seen Mr. Kelley on two separate occasions. The first visit occurred on May 5, 1999, and included your initial assessment when he filled his prescriptions. The second visit took place on June 12, 1999, almost 6 weeks later. On the second visit, you note that he is not doing peak flow monitoring at work and does not use his albuterol inhaler at work. Subsequently, he overuses his rescue inhaler after work and in the evening. Use all of this information to develop an ATAW and TPL for Mr. Kelley using the blank forms. When you have completed this assessment, compare your forms to the completed ATAW and TPL in **Appendix C**. You can go back to the information presented earlier in this module to fill in any information gaps.

Turn to the completed ATAW in Appendix C. Correlation between drug therapy and medical problems:
- No problems noted: all medications have an appropriate indication.

Appropriate therapy:
- A problem exists: patient unable to use inhaler at work.

Drug regimen:
- A problem exists: patient taking ibuprofen, may exacerbate symptoms; patient is unable to use his inhaler at work for fear of reprimand and job safety; he subsequently overuses his albuterol inhaler for rescue treatment as soon as his shift ends.

Therapeutic duplication:
- No problem exists.

Drug allergy or intolerance:
- A problem exists: Mr. Kelley reports sensitivity to aspirin; unaware of relationship to ibuprofen.

Adverse drug events:
- No problem exists.

Interactions: Drug-drug, drug-disease, drug-nutrient, drug–laboratory test:
- A problem exists: ibuprofen may exacerbate symptoms.

Social or recreational drug use:
- No problem exists.

Financial impact:
- A problem exists: Mr. Kelley does not have a prescription drug benefit.

Patient knowledge of therapy:
- A problem exists: Mr. Kelley is very anxious about his disease and wishes to learn all that he can.

Adherence:
- A problem exists; medication refill history: Mr. Kelley unable to use his medications at work.

Self-monitoring:
- No problem exists.

Risks and quality of life impacts:
- A problem exists: Mr. Kelley's job security could be jeopardized if management finds out about his asthma; he has become overly anxious and nervous about this issue, which has resulted in even poorer control of his disease.

Mr. Kelley's case is complicated because of the work-related sensitivity issue. Obviously, the pharmacist will need to work closely with Mr. Kelley to find creative ways for him to manage his disease. With the financial difficulties that are present for Mr. Kelley, you may consider contacting the manufacturer directly to see if they offer any assistance to patients that are unable to pay for expensive medications. Many companies have programs to assist individuals with financial need. Mr. Kelley is willing to learn and wants to do anything he can to both manage the disease and not lose his job. Helping Mr. Kelley find a way to control his work-related exacerbations while not financially strapping him would be the items of highest priority for Mr. Kelley. Mr. Kelley should also be counseled on his ibuprofen use because he develops shortness of breath with aspirin. If Mr. Kelley's physician wants him to take an aspirin a day for myocardial infarction prophylaxis, he will need to be desensitized to aspirin. Mr. Kelley should also be informed that he should consider getting an influenza vaccine during the next flu season.

Each asthma patient you encounter will be unique. The problem of adherence to therapy will be the most common problem you encounter. The reasons for nonadherence will depend on the age of the person, social and financial concerns, and belief that the disease needs to be and can be controlled. The ability to properly administer inhaled medications can be a challenge for both very young and elderly patients. Very young patients will most probably require the use of a spacer device, as coordinating actuation and breathing can be difficult. Elderly patients may have difficulty actuating a device because of arthritis and old age. As patients age, they often have concomitant diseases that may interfere with their asthma. Elderly patients will also be more sensitive to medications and have an increased incidence of adverse effects. Patients receiving multiple medications will have increased difficulty remembering to be adherent. Patients with multiple medications also have an increased opportunity to experience adverse reactions and drug interactions. Do not overlook these factors as you create your therapy problem lists.

Summary

In this section, we have reviewed common therapy problems associated with asthma and learned to construct a therapy problem list for ambulatory asthma patients. You will need to rely on other pharmacology and pharmacotherapeutic references for specific drug information. The information presented in this section has been provided for the purpose of building on your expert drug knowledge and formulating the information into a systematic therapy problem list for ambulatory care patients with asthma.

References

1. Schmier JK, Leidy NK. The complexity of treatment adherence in adults with asthma: challenges and opportunities [see comments]. *J Asthma* 1998;35:455–72.
2. Harrison BD. Psychosocial aspects of asthma in adults. *Thorax* 1998;53:519–25.
3. Self TH, Kelly H. Asthma. In: Young LY, Koda-Kimble MA, editors. *Applied Therapeutics: The Clinical Use of Drugs*. Vancouver, WA: Applied Therapeutics; 1995. 19-1–19-31.
4. National Heart Lung and Blood Institute. Expert Panel Report 2: Guidelines for the Diagnosis and Management of Asthma. July, 1997.

Self-Study Questions

Objective
Describe types of problems commonly present in the unreviewed therapy of ambulatory care patients with asthma.

1. Name and describe problems commonly present in the unreviewed therapy of ambulatory care patients with asthma.

Objective
Determine the presence of any of the following medication or related therapy problems in the current therapy of ambulatory care patients with asthma:
   —medication used with no medical indication;
   —medical condition for which there is no medication prescribed;
   —medication prescribed inappropriately for particular medical condition;
   —incomplete immunization status;
   —anything inappropriate in the current medication therapy regimen (dose, dosage form, schedule, duration, route of administration, method of administration);
   —presence of therapeutic duplication;
   —prescription of medication to which the patient is allergic;
   —presence or potential for adverse drug events;
   —presence or potential for clinically significant drug–drug, drug-disease, drug-nutrient, or drug–laboratory test interactions;
   —interference with medical therapy by social or cultural drug use or use of alternative therapies (e.g., herbal or homeopathic therapies);
   —problems arising from financial impact of medication therapy on the patient;
   —patient lack of understanding of medication therapy;
   —patient not adhering to medication regimen;
   —patient at risk for complications associated with asthma or another disease;
   —patient at risk because of patient-specific characteristics (e.g., age or living/working environment); or therapy is adversely impacting patient's quality of life.

2. Refer to the case of Marie Cowling in **Appendix D**. Determine what therapy problems are present for Marie.

Objective
Explain factors that are unique to ambulatory care patients with asthma to be considered when prioritizing their medication or related problems.

3. Name and explain factors that are unique to ambulatory care patients with asthma that need to be considered when prioritizing their medication or related problems.

4. Explain why adherence needs to be considered when prioritizing their medication or related problems.

5. Explain why overuse of beta$_2$-adrenergic agonists needs to be considered when prioritizing medication or related problems.

Objective
Explain special concerns in the prioritization of medication and related health care problems for ambulatory care patients with asthma.

6. Explain why therapeutic interchange can be a special concern when prioritizing medication and related health care problems for ambulatory care patients with asthma.

7. Explain why a patient's perception of his or her disease can be a special concern when prioritizing medication and related health care problems for patients with asthma.

8. Explain why overuse of beta$_2$-adrenergic agonists can be a special concern when prioritizing medication and related health care problems for ambulatory care patients with asthma.

Objective
Construct a therapy problem list for an ambulatory care patient with asthma.

9. Refer to Marie Cowling's database in **Appendix D**. Using the blank ATAW form in Appendix D, construct a therapy problem list.

Self-Study Answers

1. There are many problems that can be found in the unreviewed therapy of ambulatory care patients with asthma, including adherence issues, duplication of therapy, overuse of beta$_2$-adrenergic agonists, and inappropriate therapeutic interchange dosing of inhaled corticosteroids.

2. Overuse of beta$_2$-adrenergic agonist; no local health care provider; no PEF monitoring; possible drug-disease interaction (ibuprofen/asthma); control of arthritis pain; poor disease control.

3. Adherence factors include fear of addiction to steroids, fear that the medication won't work, fear of side effects, misconceptions about the intended use of each medication, and no plan of therapy. Duplication of therapy and overuse of beta$_2$-adrenergic agonists rather than stepping up therapy are also issues to consider.

4. Asthma is largely a self-managed disease. Adherence issues are often present. Asthma is not well controlled when adherence issues are present.

5. Overuse of beta$_2$-adrenergic agonists may signal either poorly controlled asthma or an adherence concern.

6. Inappropriate dosing changes may be present following an inhaled corticosteroid therapeutic interchange. Careful attention to ensure equipotent doses are prescribed is required to avoid under- or overdosing a patient.

7. Patients who do not perceive their disease as chronic in nature or as a threat to their overall health will be unable to understand the need for maintenance therapy for proper disease control. These patients will have difficulty with adherence to the designed therapeutic regimen.

8. Over-use of beta$_2$-adrenergic agonists signals a need to reeducate a patient and may mean that the patient will need a referral back to their primary health provider for an evaluation and perhaps a step-up in therapy.

9. When you are finished, compare your completed forms to the ones in **Appendix E**. If you find any gaps in any area of information, go back to the corresponding section in this unit or the core module.

Pharmacist's Patient Medical History Form

I. Patient Information

Name: **Jeremy Morgan**
Address: **128 Water Ave   Milford, IL   60243**
Home Phone: **222-2222**   Office Phone: _____
Date of Birth: **1-13-86**   Last year of education completed: **7th grade**
Patient lives with **Parents + sister + brother**
Caregiver (if applicable): **N/A**
Caregiver Phone: _____
Employer: **N/A**   Job Title: _____
Name of Health Insurer: **Healthy Day**
Health Ins. Card #: **11-111-111-1-03**   Social Security #: **222-22-2222**
Primary Care Physician's Name: **Dr. Lefton**   Phone: **222-3111**
Specialist Physician's Name: _____   Phone: _____
Other Health Care Practitioner: _____   Phone: _____

II. Medical History

Are you allergic to any prescription drugs or over-the-counter medications? _____
☐ Yes   ☒ No   If yes, please list the medications and type of allergic reaction experienced:
_____

Are there any medications that you are not allergic to but cannot tolerate? _____
☐ Yes   ☒ No   If yes, please list the medications and the reaction experienced:
_____

Do you use tobacco?
☐ Yes   ☒ No   If yes, what type? _____   How often? _____

Do you drink alcohol?
☐ Yes   ☒ No   If yes, what type? _____   How often? _____

Name: **Jeremy Morgan**

Please put a check (✔) next to those items listed below that apply to you:

HEART PROBLEMS	✔	URINARY/REPRODUCTIVE	✔
Chest pain (angina)		Urinary or bladder infection	
Past heart attack		Prostate problems	
Heart failure		Hysterectomy	
Irregular heartbeat		Chronic yeast infections	
Heart by-pass surgery		Kidney disease	
Rheumatic fever		Dialysis	
Other:		Other:	
EYES, EARS, NOSE & THROAT	✔	**MUSCLES AND BONES**	✔
Poor vision		Arthritis	
Poor hearing		Gout	
Glaucoma		Back problems	
Sinus problems		Amputation	
Balance disorder		Joint replacement	
Other:		Other:	
GASTROINTESTINAL	✔	**NEUROLOGICAL**	✔
Heartburn		Headaches	
Ulcer		Seizures or epilepsy	
Constipation		Parkinson's disease	
Diverticulitis		Dizziness	
Liver disease		Past stroke	
Gallbladder problems		Fainting	
Pancreatitis		Depression	
Other:		Anxiety	
		Other:	
DO YOU HAVE:	✔	**LUNG PROBLEMS**	✔
High blood pressure		Asthma	✔
Low blood pressure		Emphysema	
High cholesterol		Bronchitis	
Diabetes		Other:	
Cancer			
Anemia			
Bleeding disorder		**DO YOU HAVE OR USE …?**	✔
Hay fever		Glasses	✔
Sleeping problems		Hearing aid	
Other:		Other:	
DO YOU HAVE A FAMILY HISTORY OF:			
High blood pressure		Asthma	✔
Heart disease	✔	Other:	
Diabetes			

Name: _Jeremy Morgan_

III. CURRENT PRESCRIPTION MEDICATIONS (INCLUDING ONES RECEIVED AT OTHER PHARMACIES)

Name of prescription medicine and strength (i.e., milligrams, grams, and units)	How much do you take each time?	How many times a day do you take the medicine?	Medical problem being treated	When did you start taking this medicine?	Has the medicine helped you? Yes/No	Name of doctor or specialist who prescribed the medicine
Example: Diabeta, 2.5 mg	1	2	Diabetes	1992	Yes	Dr. Harold Smith
Azmacort	8 puffs	4 times	asthma	last year	no	Lefton
Albuterol	2 puffs	when I need it	asthma	years ago	yes	Lefton
Albuterol neb. solution	don't know	at night	asthma	years ago	yes	Lefton

IV. CURRENT NONPRESCRIPTION MEDICATIONS

Ex: ANTACIDS, ANTI-DIARRHEALS, ALLERGY MEDICINES, ANTI-NAUSEA, DIET PILLS, EAR OR EYE MEDICATIONS, LAXATIVES, PAIN RELIEVERS, VITAMINS, ETC.

Name of medicine Example: Tylenol	How often do you take it? (daily, once a week, etc.)	Name of medicine	How often do you take it?
Motrin IB	for colds		
Echinacea	daily		
Vitamin C	daily		

I certify this information is accurate and complete to the best of my knowledge. ___Jeremy Morgan___   ___3/2/99___
  signature   date

© 2000, American Society of Health-System Pharmacists, Inc. All rights reserved.

Pharmacist's Patient Database Form

Original Date: 3/6/99
Date updated: _____
Date updated: _____
Date updated: _____

Demographic and Administrative Information

Name: Jeremy Morgan	Social Security #: 222-22-2222
Address: 123 Water Ave. Milford, IL 60243	
Health Care Provider's Name: Dr. Lefton	Health Care Provider's Phone: 222-3111
Work Phone:	Home Phone: 222-2222	Date of Birth: 1-13-86
Race: White	Gender: M
Religion:	Occupation: Child (Mom = Sally)
Health Insurer: Healthy Day	Subscriber #: 11-111-111-1-03
Primary Card Holder: George Morgan	Drug Benefit: ☒ yes ☐ no copay: $ $5.00-Generic $10-Brand

Current Symptoms

Wheezing - hx of severe exacerbations & ER visits ↑ in frequency

Past Medical History

- Asthma - diagnosed @ 3 yrs
- 6 ER visits in past 12 mos.
- 4 corticosteroid bursts in 8 months

Acute and Current Medical Problems

1.
2.
3.
4.
5.
6.
7.
8.

Family/Social/Economic History

- Ø pets Ø smoking in home
- 2 sibs 8 yr ♀, 5 yr ♂

Personal Limitations

*Quit cross country team 2° asthma

Cost of medications per month $ 20.00

Allergies/Intolerances

☒ No known drug allergies

Medication	Reaction

Social Drug Use

Alcohol	Experimenting x2 mos.
Caffeine	2 cokes/day
Tobacco	Experimenting x2 mos.

Pregnancy/Breastfeeding Status

☐ Pregnant (due _____)   ☐ Breastfeeding

Diet

- ☐ Low salt — No
- ☐ Low fat — No
- ☐ Diabetic — No
- Timing of meals:

Routine Exercise/Recreation

Daily Activities/Timing

- school
- play c̄ friends
- roller blade
- bike ride

Patient Name: Jeremy Morgan

Physical Assessment/Laboratory Data—Initial/Follow-up

Date	3/6/99				
Height					
Weight	95 lbs				
Temp					
BP					
Pulse	90				
Respirations	24 (shallow)				
Peak Flow	425 l/min				
FBG					
R. Glucose					
HbA_{1c}					
T. Chol.					
LDL					
HDL					
TG					
INR					
BUN					
Cr					
ALT					
AST					
Alk Phos					
Pulse Ox	86% sat/93 pulse				

Drug Serum Concentrations

Date					

Notes:
3/6/99 – use of accessory muscles and wheezing noted on auscultation

© 2000, American Society of Health-System Pharmacists, Inc. All rights reserved.

Patient Name: Jeremy Morgan

Current Prescription Medication Regimen

Name/Dose/Strength/Route	Schedule/Frequency of Use	Indication	Start Date (and Stop Date If Applicable)	Prescriber	Adherence Issues/Efficacy
Azmacort	8 puffs QID	Asthma	May 1998	Lefton	*poor refill history
Proventil inhaler	2 puffs QID prn	Asthma	years	Lefton	*uses as needed
Proventil Nebs	0.3 ml prn	Asthma	years	Lefton	*frequently uses all night

Current Nonprescription Medication Regimen (OTC, herbal, homeopathic, nutritional, etc.)

Name/Dose/Strength/Route	Schedule/Frequency of Use	Indication	Start Date (and Stop Date If Applicable)	Prescriber	Adherence Issues/Efficacy
Motrin 200 mg	prn	Fever 2° "colds"	?	Self	
Echinacea extract	2 mL Q Day	immune booster	>1 yr	Mom	
Vitamin C 500 mg	2 tablets Q Day	immune booster	>3 yrs	Mom	

©2000, American Society of Health-System Pharmacists, Inc. All rights reserved.

Appendix A 115

Patient Name: __Jeremy Morgan__

Risk Assessment/Preventive Measures/Quality of Life

Cardiovascular Risk Assessment		
male >45 years old	1	
female >55 years old or female <55 with history of ovarectomy not taking estrogen replacement	1	
Definite MI or sudden death before age 55 year in father or male first-degree relative or before 65 year in mother or female first-degree relative [N/A]	1	
current cigarette smoking	1	
hypertension	1	
diabetes mellitus	1	
HDL cholesterol <35 mg/dl	1	
HDL cholesterol >60 mg/dl	-1	
	Total:	

Is patient at risk for complications of current conditions?   ☒ Yes   ☐ No
Specify: **Mortality 2° to asthma exacerbation**

Preventive Measures for Adults H = has been done R = patient refuses X = not applicable		Date			
Women					
Pap Smear/pelvic	Annually 19+				
Mammogram	Every 1-2Y 40-49; annually 50+				
Men					
Rectal/prostate	Annually 50+				
All Patients					
Total/HDL-C	Every 5Y 19+				
Home Fecal Occult Blood Test	Annually				
Immunizations					
Td	Every 10Y	H			
Influenza	Every fall*	Not done			
Pneumovax	Once*	Not done			

* if indicated

Quality of life issues

　　　*childhood vaccines up to date
　　　*Jeremy quit cross-country team 2° to asthma

© 2000, American Society of Health-System Pharmacists, Inc. All rights reserved.

Ambulatory Therapy Assessment Worksheet (ATAW)

Patient: Jeremy Morgan
Pharmacist: Jennifer Loudon
Date: 3/6/99

Correlation Between Drug Therapy and Medical Problems

ASSESSMENT	PRESENCE OF PROBLEM*	COMMENTS/NOTES
Any drugs without a medical indication? Any unidentified medications? Any untreated medical conditions? Do they require drug therapy?	**(1.)** A problem exists. 2. More information is needed for determination. 3. No problem exists or an intervention is not needed.	Therapy not meeting desired outcomes— Compliance issue— Overuse of beta-adrenergic agonist

Appropriate Therapy

ASSESSMENT	PRESENCE OF PROBLEM*	COMMENTS/NOTES
Comparative efficacy of chosen medication(s)? Relative safety of chosen medication(s)? Is medication on formulary? Is nondrug therapy appropriately used (e.g., diet and exercise)? Is therapy achieving desired goals or outcomes? Is therapy tailored to this patient (e.g., age, comorbid conditions, and living/working environment)?	**(1.)** A problem exists. 2. More information is needed for determination. 3. No problem exists or an intervention is not needed.	? ibuprofen causing exacerbations prolonged echinacea use

Drug Regimen

ASSESSMENT	PRESENCE OF PROBLEM*	COMMENTS/NOTES
Are dose and dosing regimen appropriate and/or within usual therapeutic range and/or modified for patient factors? Appropriateness of PRN medications (prescribed or taken that way) Is route/dosage form/mode of administration appropriate? Does regimen and length or course of therapy consider efficacy, safety, convenience, patient limitations, and cost?	**(1.)** A problem exists. 2. More information is needed for determination. 3. No problem exists or an intervention is not needed.	uses albuterol nebs all night has both albuterol nebs & inhaler

*Problem denotes any pharmacotherapeutic or related health care problem.

© 2000, American Society of Health-System Pharmacists, Inc. All rights reserved.

Therapeutic Duplication

ASSESSMENT	PRESENCE OF PROBLEM*	COMMENTS/NOTES
Any therapeutic duplication?	(1.) A problem exists. 2. More information is needed for determination. 3. No problem exists or an intervention is not needed.	albuterol nebs & inhaler

Drug Allergy or Intolerance

ASSESSMENT	PRESENCE OF PROBLEM*	COMMENTS/NOTES
Allergy or intolerance to any medications (or chemically related medications) currently being taken? Is patient using a method to alert health care providers of the allergy/intolerance or serious health problem?	1. A problem exists. 2. More information is needed for determination. (3.) No problem exists or an intervention is not needed.	

Adverse Drug Events

ASSESSMENT	PRESENCE OF PROBLEM*	COMMENTS/NOTES
Are symptoms or medical problems drug induced? What is the likelihood the problem is drug related?	1. A problem exists. 2. More information is needed for determination. (3.) No problem exists or an intervention is not needed.	

Interactions: Drug–Drug, Drug–Disease, Drug–Nutrient, Drug–Laboratory Test

ASSESSMENT	PRESENCE OF PROBLEM*	COMMENTS/NOTES
Any drug-drug interactions? Clinical significance? Any relative or absolute contraindications given patient characteristics and current/past disease states? Any drug-nutrient interactions? Clinical significance? Any drug-laboratory test interactions? Clinical significance?	(1.) A problem exists. 2. More information is needed for determination. 3. No problem exists or an intervention is not needed.	? ibuprofen causing exacerbations

*Problem denotes any pharmacotherapeutic or related health care problem.

© 2000, American Society of Health-System Pharmacists, Inc. All rights reserved.

Social or Recreational Drug Use

ASSESSMENT	PRESENCE OF PROBLEM*	COMMENTS/NOTES
Is current use of social drugs problematic? Are symptoms related to sudden withdrawal or discontinuation of social drugs?	(1.) A problem exists. 2. More information is needed for determination. 3. No problem exists or an intervention is not needed.	cigarette & alcohol experimentation

Financial Impact

ASSESSMENT	PRESENCE OF PROBLEM*	COMMENTS/NOTES
Is therapy cost-effective? Does cost of therapy represent a financial hardship for the patient?	1. A problem exists. 2. More information is needed for determination. (3.) No problem exists or an intervention is not needed.	

Patient Knowledge of Therapy

ASSESSMENT	PRESENCE OF PROBLEM*	COMMENTS/NOTES
Does patient understand the role of his/her medication(s), how to take it, and potential side effects? Would patient benefit from education tools (e.g., written patient education sheets, wallet cards, or reminder package?) Does the patient understand the role of nondrug therapy?	(1.) A problem exists. 2. More information is needed for determination. 3. No problem exists or an intervention is not needed.	Jeremy & mother unsure of medication use & role of each medication risk vs. benefit of corticosteroids needs to be addressed

Adherence

ASSESSMENT	PRESENCE OF PROBLEM*	COMMENTS/NOTES
Is there a problem with nonadherence to drug or nondrug therapy (e.g., diet and exercise)? Are there barriers to adherence or factors hindering the achievement of therapeutic efficacy?	(1.) A problem exists. 2. More information is needed for determination. 3. No problem exists or an intervention is not needed.	Refill hx: nonadherence- frequent albuterol overused

*Problem denotes any pharmacotherapeutic or related health care problem.

© 2000, American Society of Health-System Pharmacists, Inc. All rights reserved.

Self-Monitoring

ASSESSMENT	PRESENCE OF PROBLEM*	COMMENTS/NOTES
Does patient perform appropriate self-monitoring? (e.g., peak flow and blood glucose) Is correct technique employed? Is self-monitoring performed consistently, at appropriate times, and with appropriate frequency?	1. A problem exists. 2. More information is needed for determination. 3. No problem exists or an intervention is not needed.	Jeremy does not perform peak flow monitoring

Risks and Quality of Life Impacts

ASSESSMENT	PRESENCE OF PROBLEM*	COMMENTS/NOTES
Is patient at risk for complications with an existing disease state (i.e., risk factor assessment)? Is patient on track for preventive measures (e.g., immunizations, mammograms, prostate exams, eye exams)? Is therapy adversely impacting patient's quality of life? How so?	1. A problem exists. 2. More information is needed for determination. 3. No problem exists or an intervention is not needed.	Downplays need for medications—symptoms worsening. Denies severity of disease @ risk for death

other issues:

QOL is ↓ due to ↑ exacerbations

Influenza vaccine needed in the fall—frequent URIs

---

*Problem denotes any pharmacotherapeutic or related health care problem.

© 2000, American Society of Health-System Pharmacists, Inc. All rights reserved.

AMBULATORY PHARMACIST'S CARE PLAN

Patient **Jeremy Morgan** Pharmacist **Jennifer Loudon** Date **March 10, 1999**

DATE IDENTIFIED	PROBLEM (TPL)	PHARMACOTHERAPEUTIC AND RELATED HEALTH CARE GOAL	RECOMMENDATIONS FOR THERAPY	MONITORING PARAMETER(S)	DESIRED ENDPOINT(S)	MONITORING FREQUENCY
3/98	overuse of albuterol					
	intermittent refill record Azmacort					
	cigarette & alcohol use					
	self-monitoring not done					
	poor symptom recognition					
	Echinacea use for prolonged time					
	Influenza vaccine: Not vaccinated					
	Misconceptions about corticosteroids					

© 2000, American Society of Health-System Pharmacists, Inc. All rights reserved.

Pharmacist's Patient Medical History Form

I. Patient Information

Name: __Mike Kelley__
Address: __211 Clear St.   Adington, IL__
Home Phone: __111-2345__   Office Phone: __112-3456__
Date of Birth: __1-20-56__   Last year of education completed: __12th grade__
Patient lives with __spouse, 4 children (1 yr, 6 yr, 8 yr, 12 yr)__
Caregiver (if applicable): __N/A__
Caregiver Phone: __N/A__
Employer: __ACME Chemical__   Job Title: __Time Study Coordinator__
Name of Health Insurer: __Catastrophy Plan__
Health Ins. Card #: __911-911-91101__   Social Security #: __333-33-3333__
Primary Care Physician's Name: __Dr. Thompson__   Phone: __911-9111__
Specialist Physician's Name: __N/A__   Phone: ____
Other Health Care Practitioner: __N/A__   Phone: ____

II. Medical History

Are you allergic to any prescription drugs or over-the-counter medications? ____
☒ Yes   ☐ No   If yes, please list the medications and type of allergic reaction experienced:

__ASA: face swelling, difficulty breathing__

Are there any medications that you are not allergic to but cannot tolerate? ____
☐ Yes   ☒ No   If yes, please list the medications and the reaction experienced:

____

Do you use tobacco?   __smoked from 18 yrs-20 yrs (1/2 pack a day)__
☐ Yes   ☒ No   If yes, what type? ____   How often? ____

Do you drink alcohol?
☒ Yes   ☐ No   If yes, what type? __beer__   How often? __1-2 times a week__

Name: **Mike Kelley**

Please put a check (✔) next to those items listed below that apply to you:

HEART PROBLEMS	✔	URINARY/REPRODUCTIVE	✔
Chest pain (angina)		Urinary or bladder infection	
Past heart attack		Prostate problems	
Heart failure		Hysterectomy	
Irregular heartbeat		Chronic yeast infections	
Heart by-pass surgery		Kidney disease	
Rheumatic fever		Dialysis	
Other:		Other:	

EYES, EARS, NOSE & THROAT	✔	MUSCLES AND BONES	✔
Poor vision		Arthritis	
Poor hearing		Gout	
Glaucoma		Back problems	
Sinus problems		Amputation	
Balance disorder		Joint replacement	
Other:		Other:	

GASTROINTESTINAL	✔	NEUROLOGICAL	✔
Heartburn		Headaches	
Ulcer		Seizures or epilepsy	
Constipation		Parkinson's disease	
Diverticulitis		Dizziness	
Liver disease		Past stroke	
Gallbladder problems		Fainting	
Pancreatitis		Depression	
Other:		Anxiety	
		Other:	

DO YOU HAVE:	✔	LUNG PROBLEMS	✔
High blood pressure	✓	Asthma	✓
Low blood pressure		Emphysema	
High cholesterol		Bronchitis	
Diabetes		Other:	
Cancer			
Anemia			
Bleeding disorder		**DO YOU HAVE OR USE …?**	✔
Hay fever		Glasses	
Sleeping problems		Hearing aid	
Other:		Other:	

DO YOU HAVE A FAMILY HISTORY OF:			
High blood pressure	✓	Asthma	✓
Heart disease	✓	Other:	
Diabetes	✓		

Name: Mike Kelley

III. CURRENT PRESCRIPTION MEDICATIONS (INCLUDING ONES RECEIVED AT OTHER PHARMACIES)

Name of prescription medicine and strength (i.e., milligrams, grams, and units)	How much do you take each time?	How many times a day do you take the medicine?	Medical problem being treated	When did you start taking this medicine?	Has the medicine helped you? Yes/No	Name of doctor or specialist who prescribed the medicine
Example: Diabeta, 2.5 mg	1	2	Diabetes	1992	Yes	Dr. Harold Smith
Hydrochlorothiazide 25 mg	1	one	Blood Pressure	5 yrs	yes	Dr. Thompson

IV. CURRENT NONPRESCRIPTION MEDICATIONS

Ex: ANTACIDS, ANTI-DIARRHEALS, ALLERGY MEDICINES, ANTI-NAUSEA, DIET PILLS, EAR OR EYE MEDICATIONS, LAXATIVES, PAIN RELIEVERS, VITAMINS, ETC.

Name of medicine Example: Tylenol	How often do you take it? (daily, once a week, etc.)	Name of medicine	How often do you take it?
ibuprofen 200 mg	once-twice/month		

I certify this information is accurate and complete to the best of my knowledge. _Mike Kelley_   _5/5/99_
                                                                                          signature   date

© 2000, American Society of Health-System Pharmacists, Inc. All rights reserved.

Ambulatory Care Clinical Skills Program: Asthma Management — Appendix B

Pharmacist's Patient Database Form

Original Date: **5/5/99**
Date updated: _____
Date updated: _____
Date updated: _____

Demographic and Administrative Information

Name: **Mike Kelley**
Social Security #: **333-33-3333**
Address: **211 Clear Street Adington, IL 43430**
Health Care Provider's Name: **Dr. Thompson**
Health Care Provider's Phone: **911-9111**
Work Phone: **112-3456**
Home Phone: **111-2345**
Date of Birth: **1-20-56**
Race: **Black**
Gender: **M**
Religion:
Occupation: **Time Study Coordinator ACME Chemical**
Health Insurer: **Catastrophy Plan**
Subscriber #: **911-911-91101**
Primary Card Holder: **Mike Kelley**
Drug Benefit: ☐ yes ☒ no   copay: $_____

Current Symptoms

wheezing @ work ⊗ 1 month

Past Medical History

asthma as a child

Acute and Current Medical Problems

1. Hypertension
2. Asthma
3.
4.
5.
6.
7.
8.

Family/Social/Economic History

Married c̄ 4 children
father and brother had MI @ 51 and 48
mother has DM

Personal Limitations

Cost of medications per month $_____

Allergies/Intolerances

☐ No known drug allergies

Medication	Reaction
ASA	difficulty breathing

Social Drug Use

Alcohol **1-2x/week (beer)**
Caffeine
Tobacco **not currently**

Pregnancy/Breastfeeding Status

☐ Pregnant (due _____)   ☐ Breastfeeding

Diet

☐ Low salt
☐ Low fat
☐ Diabetic
Timing of meals:

Routine Exercise/Recreation

Daily Activities/Timing

© 2000, American Society of Health-System Pharmacists, Inc. All rights reserved.

Patient Name: Mike Kelley

Physical Assessment/Laboratory Data—Initial/Follow-up

	*MD office	*Pharmacy			
Date	May 5, 1999	May 5, 1999	June 12, 1999		
Height	5'10"		5'10"		
Weight	186 lbs		184 lbs		
Temp					
BP	130/80 mmHg		128/85 mmHg		
Pulse	78	80	75		
Respirations	20 wheezing shallow	15 and comfortable	15 and comfortable		
Peak Flow					
FBG					
R. Glucose					
HbA$_{1c}$					
T. Chol.					
LDL					
HDL					
TG					
INR					
BUN					
Cr					
ALT					
AST					
Alk Phos					
Hg	14				
HCT	41				
WBC	6.0				
Diff	55^S 28^B 23^L 5^M 1^E				

Drug Serum Concentrations

Date					

Notes: 5/5/98 – exam post albuterol; only occ. wheezes noted
6/12/98 – pt reports improvement c̄ meds

Patient Name: Mike Kelley

Current Prescription Medication Regimen

Name/Dose/Strength/Route	Schedule/Frequency of Use	Indication	Start Date (and Stop Date If Applicable)	Prescriber	Adherence Issues/Efficacy
Hydroclorothiazide 25 mg	1 po Q AM	HTN	x 5 yrs	Thompson	good — adherence

Current Nonprescription Medication Regimen (OTC, herbal, homeopathic, nutritional, etc.)

Name/Dose/Strength/Route	Schedule/Frequency of Use	Indication	Start Date (and Stop Date If Applicable)	Prescriber	Adherence Issues/Efficacy
ibuprofen 200 mg	200-400 mg pm	Muscle sore	2 years	—	works well

©2000, American Society of Health-System Pharmacists, Inc. All rights reserved.

Patient Name: __Mike Kelley__

Risk Assessment/Preventive Measures/Quality of Life

Cardiovascular Risk Assessment		
male >45 years old	1	
female >55 years old or female <55 with history of ovarectomy not taking estrogen replacement	1	
Definite MI or sudden death before age 55 year in father or male first-degree relative or before 65 year in mother or female first-degree relative	1	1
current cigarette smoking	1	
hypertension	1	1
diabetes mellitus	1	
HDL cholesterol <35 mg/dl	1	
HDL cholesterol >60 mg/dl	-1	
	Total:	2

Is patient at risk for complications of current conditions? ☒ Yes ☐ No
Specify: Morbidity + mortality 2° acute asthma exacerb.

Preventive Measures for Adults H = has been done R = patient refuses X = not applicable		Date				
Women		1999				
Pap Smear/pelvic	Annually 19+					
Mammogram	Every 1-2Y 40-49; annually 50+					
Men						
Rectal/prostate	Annually 50+					
All Patients						
Total/HDL-C	Every 5Y 19+	no data				
Home Fecal Occult Blood Test	Annually	R				
Immunizations						
Td	Every 10Y	H				
Influenza	Every fall*					
Pneumovax	Once*					

* if indicated

Quality of life issues
Needs Influenza vaccine

© 2000, American Society of Health-System Pharmacists, Inc. All rights reserved.

Ambulatory Therapy Assessment Worksheet (ATAW)

Patient _____
Pharmacist _____
Date _____

Correlation Between Drug Therapy and Medical Problems

ASSESSMENT	PRESENCE OF PROBLEM*	COMMENTS/NOTES
Any drugs without a medical indication? Any unidentified medications? Any untreated medical conditions? Do they require drug therapy?	1. A problem exists. 2. More information is needed for determination. 3. No problem exists or an intervention is not needed.	

Appropriate Therapy

ASSESSMENT	PRESENCE OF PROBLEM*	COMMENTS/NOTES
Comparative efficacy of chosen medication(s)? Relative safety of chosen medication(s)? Is medication on formulary? Is nondrug therapy appropriately used (e.g., diet and exercise)? Is therapy achieving desired goals or outcomes? Is therapy tailored to this patient (e.g., age, comorbid conditions, and living/working environment)?	1. A problem exists. 2. More information is needed for determination. 3. No problem exists or an intervention is not needed.	

Drug Regimen

ASSESSMENT	PRESENCE OF PROBLEM*	COMMENTS/NOTES
Are dose and dosing regimen appropriate and/or within usual therapeutic range and/or modified for patient factors? Appropriateness of PRN medications (prescribed or taken that way) Is route/dosage form/mode of administration appropriate? Does regimen and length or course of therapy consider efficacy, safety, convenience, patient limitations, and cost?	1. A problem exists. 2. More information is needed for determination. 3. No problem exists or an intervention is not needed.	

*Problem denotes any pharmacotherapeutic or related health care problem.

© 2000, American Society of Health-System Pharmacists, Inc. All rights reserved.

Therapeutic Duplication

ASSESSMENT	PRESENCE OF PROBLEM*	COMMENTS/NOTES
Any therapeutic duplication?	1. A problem exists. 2. More information is needed for determination. 3. No problem exists or an intervention is not needed.	

Drug Allergy or Intolerance

ASSESSMENT	PRESENCE OF PROBLEM*	COMMENTS/NOTES
Allergy or intolerance to any medications (or chemically related medications) currently being taken? Is patient using a method to alert health care providers of the allergy/intolerance or serious health problem?	1. A problem exists. 2. More information is needed for determination. 3. No problem exists or an intervention is not needed.	

Adverse Drug Events

ASSESSMENT	PRESENCE OF PROBLEM*	COMMENTS/NOTES
Are symptoms or medical problems drug induced? What is the likelihood the problem is drug related?	1. A problem exists. 2. More information is needed for determination. 3. No problem exists or an intervention is not needed.	

Interactions: Drug-Drug, Drug-Disease, Drug-Nutrient, Drug–Laboratory Test

ASSESSMENT	PRESENCE OF PROBLEM*	COMMENTS/NOTES
Any drug-drug interactions? Clinical significance? Any relative or absolute contraindications given patient characteristics and current/past disease states? Any drug-nutrient interactions? Clinical significance? Any drug-laboratory test interactions? Clinical significance?	1. A problem exists. 2. More information is needed for determination. 3. No problem exists or an intervention is not needed.	

*Problem denotes any pharmacotherapeutic or related health care problem.

© 2000, American Society of Health-System Pharmacists, Inc. All rights reserved.

Social or Recreational Drug Use

ASSESSMENT	PRESENCE OF PROBLEM*	COMMENTS/NOTES
Is current use of social drugs problematic? Are symptoms related to sudden withdrawal or discontinuation of social drugs?	1. A problem exists. 2. More information is needed for determination. 3. No problem exists or an intervention is not needed.	

Financial Impact

ASSESSMENT	PRESENCE OF PROBLEM*	COMMENTS/NOTES
Is therapy cost-effective? Does cost of therapy represent a financial hardship for the patient?	1. A problem exists. 2. More information is needed for determination. 3. No problem exists or an intervention is not needed.	

Patient Knowledge of Therapy

ASSESSMENT	PRESENCE OF PROBLEM*	COMMENTS/NOTES
Does patient understand the role of his/her medication(s), how to take it, and potential side effects? Would patient benefit from education tools (e.g., written patient education sheets, wallet cards, or reminder package?) Does the patient understand the role of nondrug therapy?	1. A problem exists. 2. More information is needed for determination. 3. No problem exists or an intervention is not needed.	

Adherence

ASSESSMENT	PRESENCE OF PROBLEM*	COMMENTS/NOTES
Is there a problem with nonadherence to drug or nondrug therapy (e.g., diet and exercise)? Are there barriers to adherence or factors hindering the achievement of therapeutic efficacy?	1. A problem exists. 2. More information is needed for determination. 3. No problem exists or an intervention is not needed.	

*Problem denotes any pharmacotherapeutic or related health care problem.

© 2000, American Society of Health-System Pharmacists, Inc. All rights reserved.

Self-Monitoring

ASSESSMENT	PRESENCE OF PROBLEM*	COMMENTS/NOTES
Does patient perform appropriate self-monitoring? (e.g., peak flow and blood glucose) Is correct technique employed? Is self-monitoring performed consistently, at appropriate times, and with appropriate frequency?	1. A problem exists. 2. More information is needed for determination. 3. No problem exists or an intervention is not needed.	

Risks and Quality of Life Impacts

ASSESSMENT	PRESENCE OF PROBLEM*	COMMENTS/NOTES
Is patient at risk for complications with an existing disease state (i.e., risk factor assessment)? Is patient on track for preventive measures (e.g., immunizations, mammograms, prostate exams, eye exams)? Is therapy adversely impacting patient's quality of life? How so?	1. A problem exists. 2. More information is needed for determination. 3. No problem exists or an intervention is not needed.	

*Problem denotes any pharmacotherapeutic or related health care problem.

© 2000, American Society of Health-System Pharmacists, Inc. All rights reserved.

Ambulatory Pharmacist's Care Plan

Patient _____ Pharmacist _____ Date _____

DATE IDENTIFIED	PROBLEM (TPL)	PHARMACOTHERAPEUTIC AND RELATED HEALTH CARE GOAL	RECOMMENDATIONS FOR THERAPY	MONITORING PARAMETER(S)	DESIRED ENDPOINT(S)	MONITORING FREQUENCY

AMBULATORY THERAPY ASSESSMENT WORKSHEET (ATAW)

Patient **Mike Kelley**
Pharmacist **Bob Jones**
Date **5/5/99**

Correlation Between Drug Therapy and Medical Problems

ASSESSMENT	PRESENCE OF PROBLEM*	COMMENTS/NOTES
Any drugs without a medical indication? Any unidentified medications? Any untreated medical conditions? Do they require drug therapy?	1. A problem exists. 2. More information is needed for determination. (3.) No problem exists or an intervention is not needed.	

Appropriate Therapy

ASSESSMENT	PRESENCE OF PROBLEM*	COMMENTS/NOTES
Comparative efficacy of chosen medication(s)? Relative safety of chosen medication(s)? Is medication on formulary? Is nondrug therapy appropriately used (e.g., diet and exercise)? Is therapy achieving desired goals or outcomes? Is therapy tailored to this patient (e.g., age, comorbid conditions, and living/working environment)?	(1.) A problem exists. 2. More information is needed for determination. 3. No problem exists or an intervention is not needed.	Asthma meds recently added — pt. unable to use meds @ work

Drug Regimen

ASSESSMENT	PRESENCE OF PROBLEM*	COMMENTS/NOTES
Are dose and dosing regimen appropriate and/or within usual therapeutic range and/or modified for patient factors? Appropriateness of PRN medications (prescribed or taken that way) Is route/dosage form/mode of administration appropriate? Does regimen and length or course of therapy consider efficacy, safety, convenience, patient limitations, and cost?	(1.) A problem exists. 2. More information is needed for determination. 3. No problem exists or an intervention is not needed.	ASA allergy c̄ asthma, taking ibuprofen fear of using inhaler @ work ∴ overuse of albuterol after work

*Problem denotes any pharmacotherapeutic or related health care problem.

© 2000, American Society of Health-System Pharmacists, Inc. All rights reserved.

Therapeutic Duplication

ASSESSMENT	PRESENCE OF PROBLEM*	COMMENTS/NOTES
Any therapeutic duplication?	1. A problem exists. 2. More information is needed for determination. **(3.)** No problem exists or an intervention is not needed.	

Drug Allergy or Intolerance

ASSESSMENT	PRESENCE OF PROBLEM*	COMMENTS/NOTES
Allergy or intolerance to any medications (or chemically related medications) currently being taken? Is patient using a method to alert health care providers of the allergy/intolerance or serious health problem?	**(1.)** A problem exists. 2. More information is needed for determination. 3. No problem exists or an intervention is not needed.	ASA sensitivity - ibuprofen use

Adverse Drug Events

ASSESSMENT	PRESENCE OF PROBLEM*	COMMENTS/NOTES
Are symptoms or medical problems drug induced? What is the likelihood the problem is drug related?	1. A problem exists. 2. More information is needed for determination. **(3.)** No problem exists or an intervention is not needed.	

Interactions: Drug–Drug, Drug–Disease, Drug–Nutrient, Drug–Laboratory Test

ASSESSMENT	PRESENCE OF PROBLEM*	COMMENTS/NOTES
Any drug-drug interactions? Clinical significance? Any relative or absolute contraindications given patient characteristics and current/past disease states? Any drug-nutrient interactions? Clinical significance? Any drug-laboratory test interactions? Clinical significance?	**(1.)** A problem exists. 2. More information is needed for determination. 3. No problem exists or an intervention is not needed.	ibuprofen - asthma causing symptoms - educate pt.

*Problem denotes any pharmacotherapeutic or related health care problem.

© 2000, American Society of Health-System Pharmacists, Inc. All rights reserved.

Social or Recreational Drug Use

ASSESSMENT	PRESENCE OF PROBLEM*	COMMENTS/NOTES
Is current use of social drugs problematic? Are symptoms related to sudden withdrawal or discontinuation of social drugs?	1. A problem exists. 2. More information is needed for determination. **(3.)** No problem exists or an intervention is not needed.	

Financial Impact

ASSESSMENT	PRESENCE OF PROBLEM*	COMMENTS/NOTES
Is therapy cost-effective? Does cost of therapy represent a financial hardship for the patient?	**(1.)** A problem exists. 2. More information is needed for determination. 3. No problem exists or an intervention is not needed.	Pt. does not have prescription drug benefit—financial concern is evident

Patient Knowledge of Therapy

ASSESSMENT	PRESENCE OF PROBLEM*	COMMENTS/NOTES
Does patient understand the role of his/her medication(s), how to take it, and potential side effects? Would patient benefit from education tools (e.g., written patient education sheets, wallet cards, or reminder package?) Does the patient understand the role of nondrug therapy?	**(1.)** A problem exists. 2. More information is needed for determination. 3. No problem exists or an intervention is not needed.	Pt. is anxious about disease—wishes to learn

Adherence

ASSESSMENT	PRESENCE OF PROBLEM*	COMMENTS/NOTES
Is there a problem with nonadherence to drug or nondrug therapy (e.g., diet and exercise)? Are there barriers to adherence or factors hindering the achievement of therapeutic efficacy?	**(1.)** A problem exists. 2. More information is needed for determination. 3. No problem exists or an intervention is not needed.	Pt. unable to use meds @ work

*Problem denotes any pharmacotherapeutic or related health care problem.

© 2000, American Society of Health-System Pharmacists, Inc. All rights reserved.

Self-Monitoring

ASSESSMENT	PRESENCE OF PROBLEM*	COMMENTS/NOTES
Does patient perform appropriate self-monitoring? (e.g., peak flow and blood glucose) Is correct technique employed? Is self-monitoring performed consistently, at appropriate times, and with appropriate frequency?	1. A problem exists. 2. More information is needed for determination. **(3.)** No problem exists or an intervention is not needed.	

Risks and Quality of Life Impacts

ASSESSMENT	PRESENCE OF PROBLEM*	COMMENTS/NOTES
Is patient at risk for complications with an existing disease state (i.e., risk factor assessment)? Is patient on track for preventive measures (e.g., immunizations, mammograms, prostate exams, eye exams)? Is therapy adversely impacting patient's quality of life? How so?	**(1.)** A problem exists. 2. More information is needed for determination. 3. No problem exists or an intervention is not needed.	Job security may be in jeopardy – Pt. overly anxious about disease

*Problem denotes any pharmacotherapeutic or related health care problem.

© 2000, American Society of Health-System Pharmacists, Inc. All rights reserved.

Ambulatory Pharmacist's Care Plan

Patient: Mike Kelley   Pharmacist: Bob Jones   Date: 5/5/99

DATE IDENTIFIED	PROBLEM (TPL)	PHARMACOTHERAPEUTIC AND RELATED HEALTH CARE GOAL	RECOMMENDATIONS FOR THERAPY	MONITORING PARAMETER(S)	DESIRED ENDPOINT(S)	MONITORING FREQUENCY
5/5/99	Drug-disease interaction (ibuprofen)					
	Self-monitoring					
	Needs baseline education					
	Continued symptoms					
6/12/99	Nonadherence to treatment plan					

© 2000, American Society of Health-System Pharmacists, Inc. All rights reserved.

Pharmacist's Patient Medical History Form

I. Patient Information

Name: **Marie Cowling**

Address: **220 East Sycamore   Sun City, AZ 21000**

Home Phone: **888-8888**   Office Phone: **N/A**

Date of Birth: **7-12-33**   Last year of education completed: **high school – 12th grade**

Patient lives with **Alone – recently widowed; new to area**

Caregiver (if applicable): **N/A**

Caregiver Phone: **N/A**

Employer: **Retired Receptionist**   Job Title: **–**

Name of Health Insurer: **MEDICARE**

Health Ins. Card #: **00-000-0000**   Social Security #: **444-44-4444**

Primary Care Physician's Name: **Dr. Dobson**   Phone: **630-218-4298 MD**

Specialist Physician's Name: **N/A**   Phone:

Other Health Care Practitioner: **N/A**   Phone:

II. Medical History

Are you allergic to any prescription drugs or over-the-counter medications?
☒ Yes   ☐ No   If yes, please list the medications and type of allergic reaction experienced:

Seasonal Allergies – ragweed, pollen; Erythromycin – vomits

Are there any medications that you are not allergic to but cannot tolerate?
☐ Yes   ☒ No   If yes, please list the medications and the reaction experienced:

Do you use tobacco?
☐ Yes   ☒ No   If yes, what type? _____   How often? _____

Do you drink alcohol?
☒ Yes   ☐ No   If yes, what type? **Brandy**   How often? **1/wk for sleep**

Name: **Marie Cowling**

Please put a check (✔) next to those items listed below that apply to you:

HEART PROBLEMS	✔	URINARY/REPRODUCTIVE	✔
Chest pain (angina)		Urinary or bladder infection	
Past heart attack		Prostate problems	
Heart failure		Hysterectomy 20 yrs ago	✓
Irregular heartbeat		Chronic yeast infections	
Heart by-pass surgery		Kidney disease	
Rheumatic fever		Dialysis	
Other:		Other: incontinence c̄ sneezing	✓
EYES, EARS, NOSE & THROAT	✔	**MUSCLES AND BONES**	✔
Poor vision	✓	Arthritis	✓
Poor hearing	✓	Gout	
Glaucoma		Back problems	
Sinus problems		Amputation	
Balance disorder		Joint replacement	
Other:		Other:	
GASTROINTESTINAL	✔	**NEUROLOGICAL**	✔
Heartburn		Headaches	
Ulcer		Seizures or epilepsy	
Constipation		Parkinson's disease	
Diverticulitis		Dizziness	
Liver disease		Past stroke	
Gallbladder problems		Fainting	
Pancreatitis		Depression	
Other:		Anxiety	
		Other:	
DO YOU HAVE:	✔	**LUNG PROBLEMS**	✔
High blood pressure		Asthma All of life	✓
Low blood pressure		Emphysema	
High cholesterol		Bronchitis	
Diabetes		Other: Frequent colds	
Cancer			
Anemia			
Bleeding disorder		**DO YOU HAVE OR USE …?**	✔
Hay fever		Glasses	✓
Sleeping problems		Hearing aid	
Other:		Other:	
DO YOU HAVE A FAMILY HISTORY OF:			
High blood pressure		Asthma	
Heart disease	✓	Other: Breast Cancer	✓
Diabetes			

Name: Marie Cowling

III. Current Prescription Medications (Including Ones Received at Other Pharmacies)

Name of prescription medicine and strength (i.e., milligrams, grams, and units)	How much do you take each time?	How many times a day do you take the medicine?	Medical problem being treated	When did you start taking this medicine?	Has the medicine helped you? Yes/No	Name of doctor or specialist who prescribed the medicine
Example: Diabeta, 2.5 mg	1	2	Diabetes	1992	Yes	Dr. Harold Smith
Maxair MDI	2 puffs	3	Asthma	? years	?	Dobson

IV. Current Nonprescription Medications

Ex: Antacids, anti-diarrheals, allergy medicines, anti-nausea, diet pills, ear or eye medications, laxatives, pain relievers, vitamins, etc.

Name of medicine Example: Tylenol	How often do you take it? (daily, once a week, etc.)	Name of medicine	How often do you take it?
Motrin 200 mg	2x/day (take 2 tabs)		
One-a-Day w/ calcium	1/day		

I certify this information is accurate and complete to the best of my knowledge.   Marie Cowling   7/8/99
                                                                          signature   date

© 2000, American Society of Health-System Pharmacists, Inc. All rights reserved.

Appendix D 141

Pharmacist's Patient Database Form

Original Date: **7/8/99**
Date updated: _____
Date updated: _____
Date updated: _____

Demographic and Administrative Information

Name: **Marie Cowling**	Social Security #: **444-44-4444**
Address: **220 East Sycamore Sun City, AZ**	
Health Care Provider's Name: **Dr. Dobson**	Health Care Provider's Phone: **630-218-4298**
Work Phone: **N/A** Home Phone:	Date of Birth: **7-12-33**
Race: **White**	Gender: **Female**
Religion: **N/A**	Occupation: **Retired**
Health Insurer: **MediCare**	Subscriber #: **00-000-0000**
Primary Card Holder: **Marie**	Drug Benefit: ☒ yes ☐ no copay: $ **10.00**

Current Symptoms

Breathing difficulties

Past Medical History	Acute and Current Medical Problems
hysterectomy ~20 yrs ago	1. Breathing Difficulties
Breathing problems – periodic through all of adult life	2. Allergies
Frequent colds	3. Arthritis
	4.
	5.
	6.
	7.
	8.

Family/Social/Economic History	Personal Limitations
recently widowed	None
retired	
2 children – adult; living in Minneapolis	
Moved to Sun City – 6 wks ago	

Cost of medications per month $ **20.00**

Allergies/Intolerances	Social Drug Use	
☒ No known drug allergies	Alcohol	occasional
Medication Reaction	Caffeine	None
Erythromycin GI intolerance	Tobacco	None

Pregnancy/Breastfeeding Status

☐ Pregnant (due _____)   ☐ Breastfeeding

Diet	Routine Exercise/Recreation	Daily Activities/Timing
☐ Low salt	walks 2 miles daily	
☐ Low fat		
☐ Diabetic		
Timing of meals:		

© 2000, American Society of Health-System Pharmacists, Inc. All rights reserved.

Patient Name: Marie Cowling

Physical Assessment/Laboratory Data—Initial/Follow-up

Date	7/8/99				
Height					
Weight					
Temp					
BP					
Pulse					
Respirations					
Peak Flow					
FBG					
R. Glucose					
HbA$_{1c}$					
T. Chol.					
LDL					
HDL					
TG					
INR					
BUN					
Cr					
ALT					
AST					
Alk Phos					
WBC	7.2				
Diff	85^{s}2^{8}13^L				
Pulse Ox	95%				

Drug Serum Concentrations

Date					

Notes:

Patient Name: **Marie Cowling**

Current Prescription Medication Regimen

Name/Dose/Strength/Route	Schedule/Frequency of Use	Indication	Start Date (and Stop Date If Applicable)	Prescriber	Adherence Issues/Efficacy
Maxitir MDI	2 puffs Q 8° pm	Asthma	years	Dobson	↑ frequency of use – 2 refill in 6 wks

Current Nonprescription Medication Regimen (OTC, herbal, homeopathic, nutritional, etc.)

Name/Dose/Strength/Route	Schedule/Frequency of Use	Indication	Start Date (and Stop Date If Applicable)	Prescriber	Adherence Issues/Efficacy
ibuprofen 200 mg	2 tabs BID	Arthritis	years	—	
ONE A DAY with calcium	One/day	Supplement	years	—	

©2000, American Society of Health-System Pharmacists, Inc. All rights reserved.

Patient Name: **Marie Cowling**

Risk Assessment/Preventive Measures/Quality of Life

Cardiovascular Risk Assessment		
male >45 years old	1	
female >55 years old or female <55 with history of ovarectomy not taking estrogen replacement	1	1
Definite MI or sudden death before age 55 year in father or male first-degree relative or before 65 year in mother or female first-degree relative	1	
current cigarette smoking	1	
hypertension	1	
diabetes mellitus	1	
HDL cholesterol <35 mg/dl	1	?
HDL cholesterol >60 mg/dl	-1	?
	Total:	

Is patient at risk for complications of current conditions? ☒ Yes ☐ No
Specify: Acute Exacerbation → Morbidity / Mortality

Preventive Measures for Adults
H = has been done   R = patient refuses   X = not applicable   Date

Women		2/99				
Pap Smear/pelvic	Annually 19+	X				
Mammogram	Every 1-2Y 40-49; annually 50+	H				
Men						
Rectal/prostate	Annually 50+					
All Patients						
Total/HDL-C	Every 5Y 19+	?				
Home Fecal Occult Blood Test	Annually					
Immunizations						
Td	Every 10Y	H				
Influenza	Every fall*	H				
Pneumovax	Once*	H				

* if indicated

Quality of life issues

Patient alone and fearful - breathing difficulties Controlling her life - moved to Sun City upon suggestion of MD → to improve breathing + arthritis

© 2000, American Society of Health-System Pharmacists, Inc. All rights reserved.

Ambulatory Therapy Assessment Worksheet (ATAW)

Patient _____
Pharmacist _____
Date _____

Correlation Between Drug Therapy and Medical Problems

ASSESSMENT	PRESENCE OF PROBLEM*	COMMENTS/NOTES
Any drugs without a medical indication? Any unidentified medications? Any untreated medical conditions? Do they require drug therapy?	1. A problem exists. 2. More information is needed for determination. 3. No problem exists or an intervention is not needed.	

Appropriate Therapy

ASSESSMENT	PRESENCE OF PROBLEM*	COMMENTS/NOTES
Comparative efficacy of chosen medication(s)? Relative safety of chosen medication(s)? Is medication on formulary? Is nondrug therapy appropriately used (e.g., diet and exercise)? Is therapy achieving desired goals or outcomes? Is therapy tailored to this patient (e.g., age, comorbid conditions, and living/working environment)?	1. A problem exists. 2. More information is needed for determination. 3. No problem exists or an intervention is not needed.	

Drug Regimen

ASSESSMENT	PRESENCE OF PROBLEM*	COMMENTS/NOTES
Are dose and dosing regimen appropriate and/or within usual therapeutic range and/or modified for patient factors? Appropriateness of PRN medications (prescribed or taken that way)? Is route/dosage form/mode of administration appropriate? Does regimen and length or course of therapy consider efficacy, safety, convenience, patient limitations, and cost?	1. A problem exists. 2. More information is needed for determination. 3. No problem exists or an intervention is not needed.	

*Problem denotes any pharmacotherapeutic or related health care problem.

© 2000, American Society of Health-System Pharmacists, Inc. All rights reserved.

Therapeutic Duplication

ASSESSMENT	PRESENCE OF PROBLEM*	COMMENTS/NOTES
Any therapeutic duplication?	1. A problem exists. 2. More information is needed for determination. 3. No problem exists or an intervention is not needed.	

Drug Allergy or Intolerance

ASSESSMENT	PRESENCE OF PROBLEM*	COMMENTS/NOTES
Allergy or intolerance to any medications (or chemically related medications) currently being taken? Is patient using a method to alert health care providers of the allergy/intolerance or serious health problem?	1. A problem exists. 2. More information is needed for determination. 3. No problem exists or an intervention is not needed.	

Adverse Drug Events

ASSESSMENT	PRESENCE OF PROBLEM*	COMMENTS/NOTES
Are symptoms or medical problems drug induced? What is the likelihood the problem is drug related?	1. A problem exists. 2. More information is needed for determination. 3. No problem exists or an intervention is not needed.	

Interactions: Drug-Drug, Drug-Disease, Drug-Nutrient, Drug–Laboratory Test

ASSESSMENT	PRESENCE OF PROBLEM*	COMMENTS/NOTES
Any drug-drug interactions? Clinical significance? Any relative or absolute contraindications given patient characteristics and current/past disease states? Any drug-nutrient interactions? Clinical significance? Any drug-laboratory test interactions? Clinical significance?	1. A problem exists. 2. More information is needed for determination. 3. No problem exists or an intervention is not needed.	

*Problem denotes any pharmacotherapeutic or related health care problem.

© 2000, American Society of Health-System Pharmacists, Inc. All rights reserved.

Self-Monitoring

ASSESSMENT	PRESENCE OF PROBLEM*	COMMENTS/NOTES
Does patient perform appropriate self-monitoring? (e.g., peak flow and blood glucose) Is correct technique employed? Is self-monitoring performed consistently, at appropriate times, and with appropriate frequency?	1. A problem exists. 2. More information is needed for determination. 3. No problem exists or an intervention is not needed.	

Risks and Quality of Life Impacts

ASSESSMENT	PRESENCE OF PROBLEM*	COMMENTS/NOTES
Is patient at risk for complications with an existing disease state (i.e., risk factor assessment)? Is patient on track for preventive measures (e.g., immunizations, mammograms, prostate exams, eye exams)? Is therapy adversely impacting patient's quality of life? How so?	1. A problem exists. 2. More information is needed for determination. 3. No problem exists or an intervention is not needed.	

*Problem denotes any pharmacotherapeutic or related health care problem.

© 2000, American Society of Health-System Pharmacists, Inc. All rights reserved.

Ambulatory Pharmacist's Care Plan

Patient _____ Pharmacist _____ Date _____

DATE IDENTIFIED	PROBLEM (TPL)	PHARMACOTHERAPEUTIC AND RELATED HEALTH CARE GOAL	RECOMMENDATIONS FOR THERAPY	MONITORING PARAMETER(S)	DESIRED ENDPOINT(S)	MONITORING FREQUENCY

© 2000, American Society of Health-System Pharmacists, Inc. All rights reserved.

Ambulatory Therapy Assessment Worksheet (ATAW)

Patient: **Marie Cowling**
Pharmacist: **Jim Bellows**
Date: **7/8/99**

Correlation Between Drug Therapy and Medical Problems

ASSESSMENT	PRESENCE OF PROBLEM*	COMMENTS/NOTES
Any drugs without a medical indication? Any unidentified medications? Any untreated medical conditions? Do they require drug therapy?	**(1.)** A problem exists. 2. More information is needed for determination. 3. No problem exists or an intervention is not needed.	Overuse of MaxAir— unable to exercise as desired ↑'d exacerbations

Appropriate Therapy

ASSESSMENT	PRESENCE OF PROBLEM*	COMMENTS/NOTES
Comparative efficacy of chosen medication(s)? Relative safety of chosen medication(s)? Is medication on formulary? Is nondrug therapy appropriately used (e.g., diet and exercise)? Is therapy achieving desired goals or outcomes? Is therapy tailored to this patient (e.g., age, comorbid conditions, and living/working environment)?	**(1.)** A problem exists. 2. More information is needed for determination. 3. No problem exists or an intervention is not needed.	? need for corticosteroid inhaler ? chronic sinusitis

Drug Regimen

ASSESSMENT	PRESENCE OF PROBLEM*	COMMENTS/NOTES
Are dose and dosing regimen appropriate and/or within usual therapeutic range and/or modified for patient factors? Appropriateness of PRN medications (prescribed or taken that way) Is route/dosage form/mode of administration appropriate? Does regimen and length or course of therapy consider efficacy, safety, convenience, patient limitations, and cost?	**(1.)** A problem exists. 2. More information is needed for determination. 3. No problem exists or an intervention is not needed.	

*Problem denotes any pharmacotherapeutic or related health care problem.

© 2000, American Society of Health-System Pharmacists, Inc. All rights reserved.

Therapeutic Duplication

ASSESSMENT	PRESENCE OF PROBLEM*	COMMENTS/NOTES
Any therapeutic duplication?	1. A problem exists. 2. More information is needed for determination. **(3.)** No problem exists or an intervention is not needed.	

Drug Allergy or Intolerance

ASSESSMENT	PRESENCE OF PROBLEM*	COMMENTS/NOTES
Allergy or intolerance to any medications (or chemically related medications) currently being taken? Is patient using a method to alert health care providers of the allergy/intolerance or serious health problem?	1. A problem exists. 2. More information is needed for determination. **(3.)** No problem exists or an intervention is not needed.	

Adverse Drug Events

ASSESSMENT	PRESENCE OF PROBLEM*	COMMENTS/NOTES
Are symptoms or medical problems drug induced? What is the likelihood the problem is drug related?	1. A problem exists. 2. More information is needed for determination. **(3.)** No problem exists or an intervention is not needed.	

Interactions: Drug-Drug, Drug-Disease, Drug-Nutrient, Drug–Laboratory Test

ASSESSMENT	PRESENCE OF PROBLEM*	COMMENTS/NOTES
Any drug-drug interactions? Clinical significance? Any relative or absolute contraindications given patient characteristics and current/past disease states? Any drug-nutrient interactions? Clinical significance? Any drug-laboratory test interactions? Clinical significance?	1. A problem exists. 2. More information is needed for determination. **(3.)** No problem exists or an intervention is not needed.	

*Problem denotes any pharmacotherapeutic or related health care problem.

© 2000, American Society of Health-System Pharmacists, Inc. All rights reserved.

Social or Recreational Drug Use

ASSESSMENT	PRESENCE OF PROBLEM*	COMMENTS/NOTES
Is current use of social drugs problematic? Are symptoms related to sudden withdrawal or discontinuation of social drugs?	1. A problem exists. 2. More information is needed for determination. **(3.)** No problem exists or an intervention is not needed.	

Financial Impact

ASSESSMENT	PRESENCE OF PROBLEM*	COMMENTS/NOTES
Is therapy cost-effective? Does cost of therapy represent a financial hardship for the patient?	1. A problem exists. 2. More information is needed for determination. **(3.)** No problem exists or an intervention is not needed.	

Patient Knowledge of Therapy

ASSESSMENT	PRESENCE OF PROBLEM*	COMMENTS/NOTES
Does patient understand the role of his/her medication(s), how to take it, and potential side effects? Would patient benefit from education tools (e.g., written patient education sheets, wallet cards, or reminder package?) Does the patient understand the role of nondrug therapy?	**(1.)** A problem exists. 2. More information is needed for determination. 3. No problem exists or an intervention is not needed.	↑'d use of Beta-Adrenergic Agonist

Adherence

ASSESSMENT	PRESENCE OF PROBLEM*	COMMENTS/NOTES
Is there a problem with nonadherence to drug or nondrug therapy (e.g., diet and exercise)? Are there barriers to adherence or factors hindering the achievement of therapeutic efficacy?	1. A problem exists. 2. More information is needed for determination. **(3.)** No problem exists or an intervention is not needed.	

*Problem denotes any pharmacotherapeutic or related health care problem.

© 2000, American Society of Health-System Pharmacists, Inc. All rights reserved.

Self-Monitoring

ASSESSMENT	PRESENCE OF PROBLEM*	COMMENTS/NOTES
Does patient perform appropriate self-monitoring? (e.g., peak flow and blood glucose) Is correct technique employed? Is self-monitoring performed consistently, at appropriate times, and with appropriate frequency?	(1.) A problem exists. 2. More information is needed for determination. 3. No problem exists or an intervention is not needed.	No PEF; may be helpful

Risks and Quality of Life Impacts

ASSESSMENT	PRESENCE OF PROBLEM*	COMMENTS/NOTES
Is patient at risk for complications with an existing disease state (i.e., risk factor assessment)? Is patient on track for preventive measures (e.g., immunizations, mammograms, prostate exams, eye exams)? Is therapy adversely impacting patient's quality of life? How so?	(1.) A problem exists. 2. More information is needed for determination. 3. No problem exists or an intervention is not needed.	Cannot walk as desired ↑ need for meds

*Problem denotes any pharmacotherapeutic or related health care problem.

© 2000, American Society of Health-System Pharmacists, Inc. All rights reserved.

Ambulatory Pharmacist's Care Plan

Patient __Marie Cowling__   Pharmacist __John Bellows__   Date __July 8, 1999__

DATE IDENTIFIED	PROBLEM (TPL)	PHARMACOTHERAPEUTIC AND RELATED HEALTH CARE GOAL	RECOMMENDATIONS FOR THERAPY	MONITORING PARAMETER(S)	DESIRED ENDPOINT(S)	MONITORING FREQUENCY
7/8/99	Overuse of Beta-adrenergic agonist					
	No local health care provider					
	No PEF monitoring					
	Possible drug-disease interaction					
	Improved disease control					
	Arthritis					

Appendix E 153

© 2000, American Society of Health-System Pharmacists, Inc. All rights reserved.

Pharmacist's Patient Medical History Form

I. Patient Information

Name: __Mary Franklin__

Address: __121 College Dorm Way Cowtown, USA 19776__

Home Phone: __888-7777__   Office Phone: _____

Date of Birth: __3-4-80__   Last year of education completed: __freshman year coll. – curr.__

Patient lives with __Roommate__

Caregiver (if applicable): __N/A__

Caregiver Phone: __N/A__

Employer: __N/A student__   Job Title: _____

Name of Health Insurer: __Student Health__

Health Ins. Card #: __1213489__   Social Security #: __133-33-0333__

Primary Care Physician's Name: __Dr. Faraway__   Phone: __?__

Specialist Physician's Name: __N/A__   Phone: _____

Other Health Care Practitioner: __N/A__   Phone: _____

II. Medical History

Are you allergic to any prescription drugs or over-the-counter medications? _____
☐ Yes ☒ No   If yes, please list the medications and type of allergic reaction experienced:

_____

Are there any medications that you are not allergic to but cannot tolerate? _____
☐ Yes ☒ No   If yes, please list the medications and the reaction experienced:

_____

Do you use tobacco?
☐ Yes ☒ No   If yes, what type? _____   How often? _____

Do you drink alcohol?
☒ Yes ☐ No   If yes, what type? __Beer__   How often? __2 nights/week__

Name: __Mary Franklin__

Please put a check (✔) next to those items listed below that apply to you:

HEART PROBLEMS	✔	URINARY/REPRODUCTIVE	✔
Chest pain (angina)		Urinary or bladder infection	
Past heart attack		Prostate problems	
Heart failure		Hysterectomy	
Irregular heartbeat		Chronic yeast infections	
Heart by-pass surgery		Kidney disease	
Rheumatic fever		Dialysis	
Other:		Other:	
EYES, EARS, NOSE & THROAT	**✔**	**MUSCLES AND BONES**	**✔**
Poor vision Contacts	✓	Arthritis	
Poor hearing		Gout	
Glaucoma		Back problems	
Sinus problems		Amputation	
Balance disorder		Joint replacement	
Other:		Other:	
GASTROINTESTINAL	**✔**	**NEUROLOGICAL**	**✔**
Heartburn		Headaches	
Ulcer		Seizures or epilepsy	
Constipation		Parkinson's disease	
Diverticulitis		Dizziness	
Liver disease		Past stroke	
Gallbladder problems		Fainting	
Pancreatitis		Depression	
Other:		Anxiety	
		Other:	
DO YOU HAVE:	**✔**	**LUNG PROBLEMS**	**✔**
High blood pressure		Asthma	✓
Low blood pressure		Emphysema	
High cholesterol		Bronchitis	
Diabetes		Other:	
Cancer			
Anemia			
Bleeding disorder		**DO YOU HAVE OR USE …?**	**✔**
Hay fever		Glasses	
Sleeping problems		Hearing aid	
Other:		Other:	
DO YOU HAVE A FAMILY HISTORY OF:			
High blood pressure		Asthma	
Heart disease	✓	Other:	
Diabetes			

Name: Mary Franklin

III. CURRENT PRESCRIPTION MEDICATIONS (INCLUDING ONES RECEIVED AT OTHER PHARMACIES)

Name of prescription medicine and strength (i.e., milligrams, grams, and units)	How much do you take each time?	How many times a day do you take the medicine?	Medical problem being treated	When did you start taking this medicine?	Has the medicine helped you? Yes/No	Name of doctor or specialist who prescribed the medicine
Example: Diabeta, 2.5 mg	1	2	Diabetes	1992	Yes	Dr. Harold Smith
Proventil inhaler	2-3 puffs	several	asthma	years	yes	Dr. Faraway

IV. CURRENT NONPRESCRIPTION MEDICATIONS

Ex: ANTACIDS, ANTI-DIARRHEALS, ALLERGY MEDICINES, ANTI-NAUSEA, DIET PILLS, EAR OR EYE MEDICATIONS, LAXATIVES, PAIN RELIEVERS, VITAMINS, ETC.

Name of medicine Example: Tylenol	How often do you take it? (daily, once a week, etc.)	Name of medicine	How often do you take it?
Tylenol	2 capsules – 2x/week		
ibuprofen 200 mg	2 tablets – once a month		

I certify this information is accurate and complete to the best of my knowledge. _Mary Franklin_ 9/20/99
　　signature　　　　　date

© 2000, American Society of Health-System Pharmacists, Inc. All rights reserved.

Appendix F 157

Pharmacist's Patient Database Form

Original Date: **9/20/99**
Date updated: _____
Date updated: _____
Date updated: _____

Demographic and Administrative Information

Name: **Mary Franklin**
Social Security #: **133-33-0333**
Address: **121 College Dorm Way   Cowtown, USA 19776**
Health Care Provider's Name: **Dr. Faraway**
Health Care Provider's Phone: **can't remember**
Work Phone: _____ Home Phone: **888-7777**
Date of Birth: **3/4/80**
Race: **White**
Gender: **F**
Religion: **ø**
Occupation: _____
Health Insurer: **Student Health**
Subscriber #: **1213489**
Primary Card Holder: **Mary Franklin**
Drug Benefit: ☒ yes ☐ no   copay: $ **15**

Current Symptoms

↑'d need for albuterol inhaler

Past Medical History	Acute and Current Medical Problems
Asthma since childhood	1.
	2.
	3.
	4.
	5.
	6.
	7.
	8.

Family/Social/Economic History	Personal Limitations
College Freshman	ø

Cost of medications per month $ _____

Allergies/Intolerances

☒ No known drug allergies

Medication	Reaction

Social Drug Use

Alcohol: **beer 2 nights/week - several**
Caffeine: **Pepsi - 3/day**
Tobacco: _____

Pregnancy/Breastfeeding Status

☐ Pregnant (due _____)   ☐ Breastfeeding

Diet	Routine Exercise/Recreation	Daily Activities/Timing
☐ Low salt		Classes
☐ Low fat		Aerobics - 3x/week -
☐ Diabetic		needs inhaler
Timing of meals:		

© 2000, American Society of Health-System Pharmacists, Inc. All rights reserved.

Patient Name: **Mary Franklin**

Physical Assessment/Laboratory Data—Initial/Follow-up

Date	9/20/99	10/31/99			
Height	5'4"	5'4"			
Weight	115 lbs	115 lbs			
Temp					
BP					
Pulse					
Respirations	16	14			
Peak Flow					
FBG					
R. Glucose					
HbA$_{1c}$					
T. Chol.					
LDL					
HDL					
TG					
INR					
BUN					
Cr					
ALT					
AST					
Alk Phos					

Drug Serum Concentrations

Date					

Notes: 9/20 referred to local MD (names given) for asthma eval., ↑ use of albuterol

Patient Name: __Mary Franklin__

Current Prescription Medication Regimen

Name/Dose/Strength/Route	Schedule/Frequency of Use	Indication	Start Date (and Stop Date If Applicable)	Prescriber	Adherence Issues/Efficacy
Proventil MDI	2-3 puffs 5-6x/day	wheezing	years	Dr. Faraway	*↑ use, no action plan

Current Nonprescription Medication Regimen (OTC, herbal, homeopathic, nutritional, etc.)

Name/Dose/Strength/Route	Schedule/Frequency of Use	Indication	Start Date (and Stop Date If Applicable)	Prescriber	Adherence Issues/Efficacy
Tylenol	2 tabs prn	HA	years	—	
Ibuprofen 200 mg	2 tabs prn	Cramps	years	—	

©2000, American Society of Health-System Pharmacists, Inc. All rights reserved.

Patient Name: Mary Franklin

Risk Assessment/Preventive Measures/Quality of Life

Cardiovascular Risk Assessment		
male >45 years old	1	
female >55 years old or female <55 with history of ovarectomy not taking estrogen replacement	1	
Definite MI or sudden death before age 55 year in father or male first-degree relative or before 65 year in mother or female first-degree relative	1	
current cigarette smoking	1	
hypertension	1	
diabetes mellitus	1	
HDL cholesterol <35 mg/dl	1	
HDL cholesterol >60 mg/dl	-1	-1
	Total:	-1

Is patient at risk for complications of current conditions? ☒ Yes ☐ No
Specify: Uncontrolled asthma exacerbation

Preventive Measures for Adults H = has been done R = patient refuses X = not applicable		Date				
Women		8/99				
Pap Smear/pelvic	Annually 19+	H				
Mammogram	Every 1-2Y 40-49; annually 50+					
Men						
Rectal/prostate	Annually 50+					
All Patients						
Total/HDL-C	Every 5Y 19+	H				
Home Fecal Occult Blood Test	Annually					
Immunizations						
Td	Every 10Y	H				
Influenza	Every fall*	H				
Pneumovax	Once*					

* if indicated

Quality of life issues

Pt c̄ ↑ need for Beta-adrenergic agonist; sent for eval – ? need for inhaled steroid. – will f/u in 1 wk.

AMBULATORY THERAPY ASSESSMENT WORKSHEET (ATAW)

Patient _____
Pharmacist _____
Date _____

Correlation Between Drug Therapy and Medical Problems

ASSESSMENT	PRESENCE OF PROBLEM*	COMMENTS/NOTES
Any drugs without a medical indication? Any unidentified medications? Any untreated medical conditions? Do they require drug therapy?	1. A problem exists. 2. More information is needed for determination. 3. No problem exists or an intervention is not needed.	

Appropriate Therapy

ASSESSMENT	PRESENCE OF PROBLEM*	COMMENTS/NOTES
Comparative efficacy of chosen medication(s)? Relative safety of chosen medication(s)? Is medication on formulary? Is nondrug therapy appropriately used (e.g., diet and exercise)? Is therapy achieving desired goals or outcomes? Is therapy tailored to this patient (e.g., age, comorbid conditions, and living/working environment)?	1. A problem exists. 2. More information is needed for determination. 3. No problem exists or an intervention is not needed.	

Drug Regimen

ASSESSMENT	PRESENCE OF PROBLEM*	COMMENTS/NOTES
Are dose and dosing regimen appropriate and/or within usual therapeutic range and/or modified for patient factors? Appropriateness of PRN medications (prescribed or taken that way) Is route/dosage form/mode of administration appropriate? Does regimen and length or course of therapy consider efficacy, safety, convenience, patient limitations, and cost?	1. A problem exists. 2. More information is needed for determination. 3. No problem exists or an intervention is not needed.	

*Problem denotes any pharmacotherapeutic or related health care problem.

© 2000, American Society of Health-System Pharmacists, Inc. All rights reserved.

Therapeutic Duplication

ASSESSMENT	PRESENCE OF PROBLEM*	COMMENTS/NOTES
Any therapeutic duplication?	1. A problem exists. 2. More information is needed for determination. 3. No problem exists or an intervention is not needed.	

Drug Allergy or Intolerance

ASSESSMENT	PRESENCE OF PROBLEM*	COMMENTS/NOTES
Allergy or intolerance to any medications (or chemically related medications) currently being taken? Is patient using a method to alert health care providers of the allergy/intolerance or serious health problem?	1. A problem exists. 2. More information is needed for determination. 3. No problem exists or an intervention is not needed.	

Adverse Drug Events

ASSESSMENT	PRESENCE OF PROBLEM*	COMMENTS/NOTES
Are symptoms or medical problems drug induced? What is the likelihood the problem is drug related?	1. A problem exists. 2. More information is needed for determination. 3. No problem exists or an intervention is not needed.	

Interactions: Drug-Drug, Drug-Disease, Drug-Nutrient, Drug–Laboratory Test

ASSESSMENT	PRESENCE OF PROBLEM*	COMMENTS/NOTES
Any drug-drug interactions? Clinical significance? Any relative or absolute contraindications given patient characteristics and current/past disease states? Any drug-nutrient interactions? Clinical significance? Any drug-laboratory test interactions? Clinical significance?	1. A problem exists. 2. More information is needed for determination. 3. No problem exists or an intervention is not needed.	

*Problem denotes any pharmacotherapeutic or related health care problem.

© 2000, American Society of Health-System Pharmacists, Inc. All rights reserved.

Self-Monitoring

ASSESSMENT	PRESENCE OF PROBLEM*	COMMENTS/NOTES
Does patient perform appropriate self-monitoring? (e.g., peak flow and blood glucose) Is correct technique employed? Is self-monitoring performed consistently, at appropriate times, and with appropriate frequency?	1. A problem exists. 2. More information is needed for determination. 3. No problem exists or an intervention is not needed.	

Risks and Quality of Life Impacts

ASSESSMENT	PRESENCE OF PROBLEM*	COMMENTS/NOTES
Is patient at risk for complications with an existing disease state (i.e., risk factor assessment)? Is patient on track for preventive measures (e.g., immunizations, mammograms, prostate exams, eye exams)? Is therapy adversely impacting patient's quality of life? How so?	1. A problem exists. 2. More information is needed for determination. 3. No problem exists or an intervention is not needed.	

*Problem denotes any pharmacotherapeutic or related health care problem.

© 2000, American Society of Health-System Pharmacists, Inc. All rights reserved.

Ambulatory Pharmacist's Care Plan

Patient _____ Pharmacist _____ Date _____

DATE IDENTIFIED	PROBLEM (TPL)	PHARMACOTHERAPEUTIC AND RELATED HEALTH CARE GOAL	RECOMMENDATIONS FOR THERAPY	MONITORING PARAMETER(S)	DESIRED ENDPOINT(S)	MONITORING FREQUENCY

© 2000, American Society of Health-System Pharmacists, Inc. All rights reserved.

Considering the Big Picture: Health Care Needs, Triage, and Referral

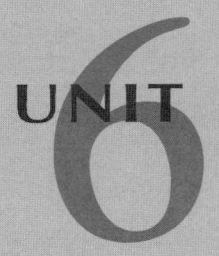
UNIT 6

Unit Objectives	166
Unit Organization	166
Health Care Needs of Ambulatory Care Patients with Asthma	166
Case Study	167
Triage and Referral of Ambulatory Care Patients with Asthma	168
Asthma Specialists	168
Mental Health Professionals	169
Social Workers	169
Urgent Situations for Ambulatory Care Patients with Asthma	169
Case Study	174
Practice Example	175
Summary	175
References	175
Self-Study Questions	176
Self-Study Answers	177

If every patient had only one health care problem, the management of that disease or symptom would be simplified. Unfortunately, most patients have multiple health care needs. The optimal treatment of an ambulatory care patient with asthma involves the formation of a partnership with the patient aimed at identifying health care needs and planning to meet those needs.

Asthma is usually a life-long disease and is associated with significant health care costs. The episodic course of asthma necessitates that at different points in the care of a patient with asthma, the partnership between the pharmacist and the patient will need to expand to draw on expertise outside the pharmacist's realm. Without a collaborative effort among members of a coordinated health care team, the patient with asthma might receive conflicting or confusing plans of care, leading to suboptimal outcomes. This collaboration should include everyone involved in the care of the patient (e.g., primary care provider, allergist, nurse practitioner, chiropractor, pharmacist, or alternative medicine professional). Every patient with asthma should have a predefined plan of action that outlines what should be done during his or her asthma exacerbations. When treating a patient with asthma, you will at times need to triage the patient based on his or her clinical state and will also need to refer a patient to another health care provider.

Unit Objectives

After you successfully complete this unit, you will be able to:
- explain factors unique to ambulatory care patients with asthma, including social and environmental factors, affecting the delivery of health care that should be considered when defining health care needs;
- define the health care needs of an ambulatory care patient with asthma;
- explain portions of the pharmacist's care plan for ambulatory care patients with asthma that should be managed by health care personnel other than pharmacists; and
- explain common situations unique to the treatment of ambulatory care patients with asthma that require immediate attention.

Unit Organization

This unit begins by discussing the health care needs of patients. We will discuss how to determine a patient's overall health care needs, using asthma as an example. We will then return to the case of Jeremy Morgan to identify his particular health care needs. Next, we will discuss the role of the ambulatory care pharmacist in the triage of patients with asthma, not only in the emergency situation but also in the management of other identified health care needs. Finally, we will discuss the development of a patient-specific emergency identification and action plan.

Health Care Needs of Ambulatory Care Patients with Asthma

Asthma is characterized in most patients by periods of stability accentuated by episodes of increased morbidity. Patients with asthma will have different health care needs at each interaction with the pharmacist. These needs will depend on the disease process as well as other life issues. A pharmacist caring for patients with asthma will need to be able to rapidly assess a patient's health care needs.

Unit 11 of the *Ambulatory Care Clinical Skills Program: Core Module* provides an excellent discussion of the process of defining health care needs. It defines three basic goals of caring for patients:
- to identify all actual or potential health care problems,
- to alleviate actual problems, and
- to avoid potential problems.

These goals also form a foundation for caring for patients with asthma and place the patient, rather than the disease, at the center of your assessment. With these goals in mind, you will be equipped to take care of the whole patient.

The prevention or reduction of chronic and troublesome symptoms requires the identification of those symptoms. Asthma presents differently with each patient. It will be necessary for the patient and the pharmacist to identify symptoms the patient may consider normal. As a health care provider, you will recognize the seriousness of these same symptoms. It is also necessary to allow the patient to identify symptoms he or she feels most affect daily activities. Recognize that both sets of symptoms are important as you identify and address patient needs and expectations. Adherence to prescribed therapies may be enhanced when patient expectations are met.[1]

Asthma costs contribute significantly to the overall costs of health care. As mentioned in unit 1, a significant portion of these costs is associated with emergent exacerbations of the disease. Treatment of patients with emergent exacerbations of asthma also significantly increases their interaction with the health care system, and disjointed care may result if patients do not feel empowered and in control of their disease. Each uncoordinated intervention by the health care system can result in a change in the patient's treatment plan without full understanding by the patient or other members of the health care team. In some cases, patients may have emergency room physicians as their primary health care providers.

Asthma can be expensive for individuals as well. Medications and monitoring devices may be required on a chronic basis. Pharmacists must understand the financial implications of therapy decisions for their patients to avoid financial barriers to adherence with a treatment plan. Inability to afford needed medications or monitoring devices may lead to increased emergency room visits for treatment. Referring a patient to a social worker may be necessary when financial constraints place the patient at high risk for nonadherence and adverse outcomes.

Patients with asthma may experience exacerbations of their disease at any time. The patient with asthma needs to be able to contact members of the health care team and obtain needed medications outside normal business hours. Where there are large populations of asthma patients, you may need to consider extending your clinic or pharmacy hours. When extension of hours is not an option, providing the patient with a list of after-hours resources for medication needs, questions, or evaluation will be an important component of care. Use of an action plan with gradated steps to take in case of worsening symptoms should reduce the need for after-hours or urgent evaluation. Part of your job will be to educate the patient and help him or her understand what to do at the first sign of an exacerbation, increased symptoms, or difficulty breathing.

The health care needs for each asthma patient will most likely vary with each pharmacist-patient encounter. Identification of health care needs, however, will provide the framework for interventions that may be required.

Case Study

Let's return to the case of Jeremy Morgan. What are his health care needs? In unit 1 you learned that he is an adolescent patient with a significant history of asthma. His mother is concerned that his disease is getting worse. You have recorded the information from Mrs. Morgan on the Pharmacist's Patient Database Form (unit 5, Appendix A).

From the patient interview you discover that Jeremy does not have a good understanding of his symptoms or of asthma itself. You had to encourage him to use his rescue inhaler during your physical exam. You also discovered that he is not using his medications appropriately. You ascertained that he has significant nighttime symptoms. He has had increased emergency room visits over the past several years.

With the data that you have collected you are able to determine that Jeremy's asthma is not well controlled. The ATAW and TPL list several problems that exist with his current drug therapy regimen.

After identifying Jeremy's current health status and the elements of care needed to improve it or prevent its deterioration, the following health care needs can be determined:
- maintenance of normal pulmonary function,
- management of disease to restore ability to participate in athletics at school,
- prevention of nocturnal symptoms,
- reduction or elimination of emergency room visits,
- avoidance of adverse medication effects, and
- improvement of patient adherence to drug and nondrug therapy.

In addition, Jeremy needs to identify triggers for his exacerbations and develop a plan for avoiding those triggers or increasing prophylaxis during times of exposure. Routine preventive care is important for all patients with a chronic disease. Two additional health care needs for Jeremy can be identified:
- identification of triggers, and
- adherence with yearly influenza vaccination.

Triage and Referral of Ambulatory Care Patients with Asthma

The pharmacist managing the care of a patient with asthma will find many instances requiring triage and referral. The episodic nature of the disease requires the expertise of additional health care professionals at different points. Lifestyle changes will affect health care needs and will necessitate triage and referral.

The patient benefits most from well coordinated care, which requires all members of a patient's health care team to communicate on a regular basis. Pharmacists practicing in ambulatory care settings should share their information with other members of the team, assuming the patient (or caregiver) has given his or her permission. As discussed in unit 12 of the *Core Module*, this communication should be in a written format.

Referrals to other health care providers should be made as formal communications. Copies of these referrals should be kept with the patient's database. Follow-up with the patient about the referral should be done on a routine basis to identify changes in the patient's overall management. At times in the treatment of the patient with asthma, the pharmacist will not be in a position to make the referral. Instead, the pharmacist will provide the patient and/or primary health care provider with additional information that supports a referral outside the patient's current health care team.

Asthma Specialists

The treatment of most patients with asthma is conducted adequately by primary care providers. Certain patients benefit from referral to an asthma specialist, usually either a pulmonologist or fellowship-trained allergist. The additional training of asthma specialists may help them uncover confounding factors in a patient's disease. The National Heart, Lung, and Blood Institute Expert Panel Report 2 contains guidelines (summarized in **Table 1**) for referral to an asthma specialist.[2] Pharmacists should be familiar with these guidelines and use them to educate patients and their primary care providers, as necessary. In many health plans referral to a specialist is not encouraged. Partnering with the primary care provider and using the national guidelines as a

Table 1. Guidelines for Referring a Patient to an Asthma Specialist

Patient has had a life-threatening asthma exacerbation.

Patient is not meeting the goals of asthma therapy after 3 to 6 months of treatment (an earlier referral or consultation is appropriate if the physician concludes that the patient is unresponsive to therapy).

Signs and symptoms are atypical or there are problems in differential diagnosis.

Other conditions complicate asthma or its diagnosis (e.g., chronic sinusitis, gastrointestinal reflux, or chronic obstructive pulmonary disease).

Additional diagnostic testing is indicated.

Patient requires additional education and guidance.

Patient is being considered for immunotherapy.

Patient has severe persistent asthma, requiring step 4 care.

Patient requires continuous oral corticosteroid therapy or high-dose inhaled corticosteroids or has required more than two bursts of oral corticosteroids in 1 year.

Patient is under age 3 and requires step 3 or 4 care.

Patient requires confirmation that an occupational or environmental inhalant is contributing to asthma.

Source: adapted with permission from reference 2.

reference may facilitate either a referral or a change in therapy that is in accord with the suggested Expert Panel Report 2 guidelines. Although the Expert Panel Report 2 guidelines have been available since February 1997, not everyone is aware of them. Part of your job will be to help familiarize other health care providers with these guidelines.

Mental Health Professionals

In treating ambulatory care patients with asthma, you will encounter patients with significant psychiatric, psychosocial, or family problems that interfere with their ability to follow a treatment plan. These patients may benefit from additional interventions provided by mental health professionals.[2] As with referral to an asthma specialist, the use of mental health services may require specialized referral and the patient may incur additional expenses. These concerns must be weighed against the benefits that the referral may bring to the patient's asthma management. The partnership of the ambulatory care pharmacist with the primary care provider will be necessary to facilitate these referrals.

Social Workers

The social worker has a pivotal role in the treatment of some asthma patients. Maneuvering within the health care system is beyond the capabilities of many patients with asthma. This inability can lead to increased use of emergency rooms as the main source of asthma care. A social worker can help a patient obtain a primary care provider who is local, has hours of operation that meet the patient's needs, and who is within the patient's health care plan. A social worker can also facilitate home visits to identify environmental or social factors that may be contributing to a patient's disease course. Social workers may also be needed, as discussed in unit 5, to assist in the coordination of care for pediatric patients.

Urgent Situations for Ambulatory Care Patients with Asthma

Triage of an ambulatory care patient with asthma includes assessment of the urgency of the situation. As described in unit 12 of the *Core Module*, urgency is influenced by:
- the patient's age,
- the type and severity of symptoms,
- the length and course of illness, and
- the patient's other medical conditions.

The Expert Panel Report 2 suggests that patients with moderate-to-severe persistent asthma and patients with a history of severe exacerbations have a written action plan. This plan needs to address patient actions in the event of worsening symptoms and exacerbations.[2] The action plan is individualized for each patient and describes how to adjust medications in response to particular signs, symptoms, and peak flow measurements. The patient should understand and accept the action plan. All members of the health care team should also be aware of the action plan. In the case of pediatric patients, parents, caregivers, school nurses, and coaches should all be aware of the action plan. For adult patients, family members and significant others should be included in discussions of the action plan. Communication before the development of an urgent situation will facilitate orchestration of the optimal course for the patient, rather than confounding the situation by over- or under-recognition of the emergent nature of the occurrence. In addition, all patients with asthma should understand the symptoms of their disease that require medical intervention. Sample action plans are provided in **Figure 1**.

Pharmacists caring for patients with asthma should recognize signs and symptoms that will require treatment. The pharmacist should also form a partnership with the primary care provider to understand his or her comfort levels with specific urgent referral parameters. Symptoms that should raise a red flag to the pharmacist include:
- inability to talk or complete a sentence,
- inability to move air on physical exam,
- signs of cyanosis, and
- complaints of nonresponse to medication.

These are not the only indications of an urgent situation. The Expert Panel Report 2 encourages practitioners to be familiar with the characteristics of asthma patients at risk for life-threatening deterioration (**Tables 2 and 3**).[2] These patients should receive aggressive treatment when exacerbations start. Remember that at times you may be assessing the patient over the telephone. Your only information might be that a patient is having a difficult time talking or breathing.

Triage and referral are especially important in the management of asthma. As a pharmacist you may be the first person to recognize an acute exacerbation, worsening disease, chronic adherence problems, or the need for intervention. The level of intervention necessary will depend on the patient's symptoms. Some of these interventions

ASTHMA ACTION PLAN (EXAMPLE 1)

Name _____ Date _____

It is important in managing asthma to keep track of your symptoms, medications, and Peak Expiratory Flow (PEF). You can use the colors of a traffic light to help learn your asthma medications:

A. **GREEN means Go** Use preventive (anti-inflammatory) medicine.
B. **YELLOW means Caution** Use quick-relief (short-acting bronchodilator) medicine in addition to the preventive medicine.
C. **RED means STOP!** Get help from a doctor.

A. Your GREEN ZONE is _____ 80 to 100% of your personal best. **GO!**
   Breathing is good, with no cough, wheeze, or chest tightness during work, school, exercise, or play.

   ACTION:
   ❑ Continue with medications listed in your daily treatment plan.

B. Your **YELLOW ZONE** is _____ 50 to less than 80% of your personal best. **CAUTION!**
   Asthma symptoms are present (cough, wheeze, chest tightness).
   Your peak flow number drops below _____ or you notice:
   ❑ Increased need for inhaled quick-relief medicine
   ❑ Increased asthma symptoms upon awakening
   ❑ Awakening at night with asthma symptoms
   ❑ _____

   ACTIONS:
   ❑ Take _____ puffs of your quick-relief (bronchodilator) medicine _____.
      Repeat _____ times.
   ❑ Take _____ puffs of _____ (anti-inflammatory) _____ times/day.
   ❑ Begin/increase treatment with oral corticosteroids.
   ❑ Take _____mg of _____ every _____ a.m. _____ p.m.
   ❑ Call your doctor (phone) _____ or emergency room _____.

C. Your **RED ZONE** is _____ 50% or less of your personal best. **DANGER!!**
   Your peak flow number drops below _____, or you continue to get worse after increasing treatment according to the directions above.

   ACTIONS:
   ❑ Take _____ puffs of your quick-relief (bronchodilator) medicine _____.
      Repeat _____ times.
   ❑ Begin/increase treatment with oral corticosteroids. Take _____ mg now.
   ❑ Call your doctor now (phone _____). If you cannot contact your doctor, go directly to the emergency room (phone _____).
   ❑ Other important phone numbers for transportation _____ .

   AT ANY TIME, CALL YOUR DOCTOR IF:
   ❑ Asthma symptoms worsen while you are taking oral corticosteroids, or
   ❑ Inhaled bronchodilator treatments are not lasting 4 hours, or
   ❑ Your peak flow number remains or falls below _____ in spite of following the plan.

Physician Signature _____ Patient/Family Member's Signature _____

Figure 1. Sample action plans (reprinted from reference 2).

ASTHMA ACTION PLAN (EXAMPLE 2)

Asthma Action Plan

Name: _____
Doctor's Name: _____
Doctor's Phone: _____
Baseline/Personal Best Peak Flow: _____
Medicines: _____
_____

ZONE	ACTIONS
Green	
Yellow	
Red	

Source: adapted with permission from Cecilia Vicuña-Kneady, R.N., in reference 2.

ASTHMA ACTION PLAN (EXAMPLE 3)

Adult Self-Management Instructions for Asthma Action Plan

Date_____.

When to Monitor Peak Flow Numbers	*Important Peak Flow Numbers*
❏ In the morning soon after waking up.	Baseline_____.
❏ Before supper.	_____% baseline_____.
❏ Before bed.	_____% baseline_____.
❏ Before and 5–15 minutes after inhaled treatments.	
❏ With increased respiratory symptoms.	
❏ _____.	

If your peak flow number drops below_____ or you notice:
- Increased use of inhaled treatments to manage asthma
- Increased asthma symptoms upon awakening
- Awakening at night with asthma symptoms
- _____.

Follow these treatment steps:
- ❏ Increase inhaled corticosteroids.
 Take_____puffs of_____times a day.
- ❏ Begin/increase treatment with oral corticosteroids.
 Take_____mg of_____.
 In the ❏ morning and/or ❏ before supper.
- ❏ _____.

If your peak flow number drops below_____ or you continue to get worse after increasing treatment according to the directions above, follow these treatment steps:
- ❏ Begin/increase treatment with oral corticosteroids.
 Take_____mg of_____.
 In the ❏ morning and/or ❏ before supper.
 Contact your health care provider.

Contact your health care provider if:
- ❏ Asthma symptoms worsen while you are taking oral corticosteroids or,
- ❏ Inhaled bronchodilator treatments are not lasting 4 hours or,
- ❏ Your peak flow number falls below_____.
- ❏ If you cannot contact your health care provider go directly to the Emergency Room.

Directions for Resuming Normal Treatment:
- ❏ Continue increased treatment until symptoms and peak flow number have returned to normal, then continue increased inhaled corticosteroids or_____mg of oral corticosteroids for the same number of days it took to return to normal. If your peak flow number has not returned to normal in 5 days contact your health care provider.
- ❏ Call your health care provider for specific instructions.

If you have questions please call:
- ❏ _____ ❏ Other _____ After hours
- ❏ Your home physician.

Physician Signature _____ Date _____

Patient/Family Signature _____ Staff Signature _____

ASTHMA ACTION PLAN (PEAK FLOW MONITORING)

Zone	Level	Status	Action
Green Zone: All Clear My best peak flow: _____ Peak Flow: _____ to _____ (100–80% of My Best Peak Flow) • No symptoms of an asthma episode • Able to do usual activities • Usual medications control asthma	**1**	**DOING WELL**	**TAKE:** Medicine _____ Dose _____ Max # times/day _____
Yellow Zone: Caution Peak Flow: _____ to _____ (80–50% of My Best Peak Flow) • Increased asthma symptoms (including wakening at night due to asthma) • Usual activities somewhat limited • Increased need for asthma medications	**2**	**INCREASE IN SYMPTOMS**	**ADD:** Medicine _____ Dose _____ Max # times/day _____ Return to Level 1 when symptoms improve
Red Zone: Medical Alert Peak Flow: Less than _____ (50% of My Best Peak Flow) • Increased symptoms longer than 24 hrs • Very short of breath • Usual activities severely limited • Asthma medications haven't reduced symptoms	**3**	**NO IMPROVEMENT AFTER ___ HRS** OR **EVEN MORE SYMPTOMS**	**ADD:** Medicine _____ Dose _____ AND CALL YOUR HEALTH CARE PROVIDER ☞ Go to the hospital *now* ☞ or Call 911 *now*

DANGER SIGNS: Difficulty walking and talking due to shortness of breath
Lips or fingernails are blue

Table 2. Risk Factors for Death from Asthma

- Past history of sudden severe exacerbations
- Prior intubation for asthma
- Prior admission for asthma to an intensive care unit
- Two or more hospitalizations for asthma in the past year
- Three or more emergency care visits for asthma in the past year
- Hospitalization or an emergency care visit for asthma within the past month
- Use of >2 canisters per month of inhaled short-acting beta$_2$-adrenergic agonist
- Current use of or recent withdrawal from systemic corticosteroids
- Difficulty perceiving airflow obstruction or its severity
- Comorbidity, as from cardiovascular disease or chronic obstructive pulmonary disease
- Serious psychiatric disease or psychosocial problems
- Low socioeconomic status and urban residence
- Illicit drug use
- Sensitivity to *Alternaria*

Source: reprinted from reference 2.

Table 3. Special Considerations for Infants

- Assessment depends on physical examination rather than objective measurements. Use of accessory muscles, paradoxical breathing, cyanosis, and a respiratory rate >60 are key signs of serious distress.
- Objective measurements such as oxygen saturation of <91 percent also indicate serious distress.
- Response to beta$_2$-adrenergic agonist therapy can be variable and may not be a reliable predictor of satisfactory outcome. However, because infants are at greater risk for respiratory failure, a *lack* of response noted by either physical examination or objective measurements should be an indication for hospitalization.
- Use of oral corticosteroids early in the episode is essential but not substitute for careful assessment by a physician.
- Most acute wheezing episodes result from viral infections and may be accompanied by fever. Antibiotics are generally not required.

will be within the scope of your practice; others will require a referral. Patients in severe distress may need to have an ambulance called for them. Other patients may simply need to be reminded to use their rescue medications. Other interventions may be as simple as recognizing nonadherence to an inhaled corticosteroid or overuse of a beta$_2$-adrenergic agonist. In these cases, you have the opportunity to educate the patient and contact his or her primary care provider to provide an update on significant findings. For example, a patient who is not on a chronic anti-inflammatory agent but is overusing short-acting beta$_2$-adrenergic agonists may need to be referred to his or her primary care provider for addition of an anti-inflammatory agent.

Case Study

Consideration of further referral of a patient should include assessment of whether any interventions have already been attempted. Consider Jeremy Morgan, who presented for his initial patient interview in respiratory distress. The pharmacist counseled Jeremy on his current symptoms and encouraged Jeremy to use his rescue treatment. Had the pharmacist ascertained that Jeremy had already administered one dose of his bronchodilator, a referral to the emergency room might have been warranted.

After he counseled Jeremy to use his bronchodilator, the pharmacist continued with his evaluation and completed the database form. From the information you gather, can you identify any referrals that should be made?

The pharmacist was able to identify some gaps in the understanding of both Jeremy and his mother about asthma management, beginning with early recognition of signs and symptoms of distress. The pharmacist noted that Jeremy's primary mode of asthma management was multiple emergency room visits. The first referral you should make is to the primary care provider. You will need to obtain permission from the patient and his mother to share information you have gathered with the primary care provider. Once permission has been obtained, you should outline the information you have gathered from the patient and his mother. You can outline educational interventions you will initiate with Jeremy and his mother. You should communicate with the physician the patient's lack of understanding about the management of exacerbations and the severity of nighttime symptoms that Jeremy has described to you.

Practice Example

It's your turn to practice. Let's return to the case of Mr. Kelley. What are his health care and triage/referral needs at this time?
- minimize symptoms related to his disease
- identify and minimize exposure to his trigger(s)
- maintain his current job

You already referred Mr. Kelley to his primary care provider. At this time, no further referrals are necessary. You will need to follow Mr. Kelley's course closely over the next few weeks to determine whether additional referrals are warranted. He may ultimately need the services of a social worker, because his current employer's health insurance is only catastrophic and does not provide medication coverage or outpatient visits. The social worker may also be helpful in the event that Mr. Kelley wishes to discuss his job security concerns.

Summary

Pharmaceutical care embraces the whole patient. The identification of each patient's unique health care needs is an essential component in the development of a pharmaceutical care plan for an ambulatory care patient with asthma. Pharmacists caring for patients with asthma must be able to triage each patient based on these identified needs as well as refer patients to other members of the health care team when appropriate.

References

1. Burke LE, Dunbar-Jacob J. Adherence to medication, diet, and activity recommendations: from assessment to maintenance. *J Cardiovasc Nurs* 1995;9:62–79.
2. National Heart, Lung, and Blood Institute. Expert Panel Report 2: Guidelines for the Diagnosis and Management of Asthma. July 1997.

Self-Study Questions

Objective
Explain factors unique to ambulatory care patients with asthma, including social and environmental factors, affecting the delivery of health care that should be considered when defining their health care needs.

1. Why should the patient's ability to identify symptoms of his or her disease be considered when defining health care needs for an ambulatory care patient with asthma?

2. Explain the effect of costs on the delivery of health care that should be considered when defining health care needs for ambulatory care patients with asthma.

3. Explain the impact of hours of care on the delivery of health care that should be considered when defining health care needs for ambulatory care patients with asthma.

Objective
Define the health care needs of an ambulatory care patient with asthma.

4. Recall the patient Marie Cowling (unit 5, appendixes D and E). Define her health care needs at this time.

Objective
Explain portions of the pharmacist's care plan for ambulatory care patients with asthma that should be managed by health care personnel other than pharmacists.

5. Explain why psychosocial issues should be managed by health care personnel other than pharmacists.

6. Explain why a patient who has had a life-threatening exacerbation should be referred to an asthma specialist.

7. Explain why a patient unable to secure treatment within the health care system should be referred to a social worker.

Objective
Explain common situations unique to the treatment of patients with asthma that require immediate attention.

8. Name and describe common situations unique to treatment of patients with asthma that require immediate attention.

Self-Study Answers

1. Patients and health care professionals may perceive the severity of symptoms differently. Symptoms a health care professional would consider serious may have plagued a patient for such a long time they are considered normal by the patient. There may be other symptoms that the patient considers to be serious. The ability to identify symptoms will affect the patient's action plan.

2. Costs associated with asthma care on a societal as well as an individual basis are significant. Patients must be able to acquire the necessary medications and monitoring devices to adequately manage their disease. If this need is not met it can lead to an inability to adhere to the treatment plan and can result in more frequent use of emergency rooms.

3. Asthma is an episodic disease. The timing of exacerbations is unpredictable in most instances. Professionals caring for patients with asthma should provide for coverage throughout as much of the day as possible. Patients should have clear directions in their action plan of how to get additional medications, if needed, as well as access care during nontraditional hours.

4. Marie Cowling's identified health care needs at this time include:
   - minimization of symptoms,
   - location of a health care provider locally, and
   - optimization of drug regimen.

   Marie is reporting that symptoms have increased in frequency, prompting her family physician to suggest a move to a different climate. Marie's symptoms have continued despite the move. She is very dependent on her $beta_2$-adrenergic agonist. A local health care provider is essential for Marie to provide support and treatment options to improve her functional status.

5. Patients with underlying psychosocial issues may have difficulty understanding or following a treatment plan.

6. The asthma specialist has training beyond the general practitioner and may be able to identify other confounding variables that might have led to the life-threatening event.

7. The social worker has expertise in the health care system and can help a patient navigate through the system. Patients unable to maneuver through the system efficiently frequently resort to the emergency room.

8. Symptoms that require immediate attention include the inability of a patient to talk or complete a sentence, the inability of a patient to move air on physical exam, signs of cyanosis, and a lack of response to medication.

Identifying Pharmacotherapeutic and Related Health Care Goals for Asthma Patients

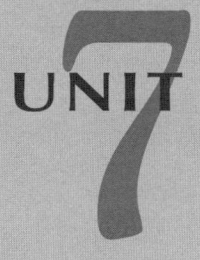

UNIT 7

Unit Objectives	180
Unit Organization	180
Factors to Consider When Identifying Pharmacotherapeutic and Related Health Care Goals	180
Disease Characteristics of Asthma	180
Health Care Goals of Other Health Care Professionals	181
Drug Therapy Problems	181
Patient-Related Factors	182
Quality of Life	182
Ethical Issues	183
The Role of Ambulatory Care Patients with Asthma in Determining Their Goals	183
Health Beliefs	183
Motivation	184
Adherence	184
Case Study	184
Realistic Treatment Outcomes for Ambulatory Care Patients with Asthma	185
Example Case	186
Practice Example	187
Summary	187
References	187
Self-Study Questions	188
Self-Study Answers	189
Appendixes	190

The identification of problems for a patient's Therapy Problem List (TPL) and identification of health care needs are the basis of the pharmaceutical care plan you will develop for the patient. The next step you will take is the establishment of pharmacotherapeutic and related health care goals. The goals you choose for each patient will be unique and will take into consideration all you have learned about the patient. Goals should be developed in collaboration with the patient. These goals are the expected pharmacotherapeutic and health-related outcomes of therapy. Defining these goals will be the focus of this unit.

Unit Objectives

After you successfully complete this unit, you will be able to:
- explain factors unique to ambulatory care patients with asthma that may influence decisions about pharmacotherapeutic and related health care goals, including:
  - disease characteristics of asthma,
  - common goals of other health care professionals,
  - common drug therapy problems,
  - patient-related factors,
  - quality-of-life issues, and
  - ethical issues;
- explain the role of ambulatory care patients with asthma in determining their therapy goals;
- explain realistic limits of treatment outcomes for patients with asthma in the ambulatory care setting; and
- specify pharmacotherapeutic and related health care goals for an ambulatory care patient with asthma that integrate patient-specific data, disease-specific and medication-specific information, and ethical and quality-of-life considerations.

Unit Organization

This unit begins with a brief discussion of issues patients with asthma may face and the influence these issues have on the establishment of treatment goals. The role of the patient with asthma in determining goals is then discussed. Finally, cases will be presented to offer additional practice in identifying goals for patients with asthma.

Factors to Consider When Identifying Pharmacotherapeutic and Related Health Care Goals

Disease Characteristics of Asthma

The natural course of asthma is a significant factor to consider when setting goals. It will dictate the drug and nondrug therapies you recommend for patients as well as contribute to the establishment of a monitoring plan.

Unit 13 of the *Ambulatory Care Clinical Skills Program: Core Module* reviews three questions that must be asked when assessing the goals for disease control:
- Is this disease acute or chronic?
- Is this disease amenable to nondrug therapy alone or is drug therapy required?
- What previous therapies has the patient received and were they successful?

Asthma is a disease characterized by periods of exacerbations and of relative stability. In considering the first of the questions above, the answer for asthma may be yes to both responses. Asthma is a chronic disease that may require continuous treatment in some patients. Acute exacerbations require urgent attention and will have different treatment and goals. The episodic course of asthma affects the ability of many patients to adhere to a regimen during periods of stability. The severity of asthma that a patient presents with is also important when defining pharmacotherapeutic and related health care goals. The severity will dictate the types of interventions that are made as well as the goals that are set by you and the patient.

According to the National Heart, Lung, and Blood Institute Expert Panel Report 2 (Expert Panel Report 2), goals for care of a patient diagnosed with asthma include[1]:
- prevention of chronic and troublesome symptoms,
- maintenance of (near) normal pulmonary function,
- maintenance of normal activity levels (including exercise and other physical activity),
- prevention of recurrent exacerbations of asthma and avoidance of emergency department visits or hospitalizations,

- provision of optimal pharmacotherapy with minimal or no adverse effects, and
- fulfillment of patients' and families' expectations of asthma care and assurance of their satisfaction with it.

It is important to have these goals in mind as you identify health care needs. The achievement of these goals necessitates identification of each patient's unique health care needs.

Consider the first time that you interact with Jeremy Morgan. He has both acute and chronic health care needs related to his asthma. Acutely, he needs relief from the symptoms he is experiencing in order to improve air exchange. He also appears to need support in managing his disease on a chronic basis, understanding the importance of monitoring and symptom recognition, as well as understanding the need for adherence to prescribed therapy.

Health Care Goals of Other Health Care Professionals

As you design your pharmacist's care plan for a patient, it will be important to identify not only the patient's goals but also the goals of other members of the patient's health care team. Without communication between health care providers, the goals the patient is expected to meet may be confusing and even conflicting. You must remember that if the patient is expected to carry the ball on the team, he or she must be working from a single playbook. All the coaches, including parents, significant others, sports coaches, school or daycare providers, and health care professionals, must use the same playbook.

As you and a patient determine goals, it is also important that you share those goals with other members of the health care team. Just as you need their information, other members of the patient's health care team will need the information you gather and the plan you formulate in order to best support the patient in attaining the goals that you and the patient have set.

Let's consider a patient, Joe Ferguson, who is managed by an internist and a chiropractor with whom he has had a long-standing relationship. The chiropractor tells Joe that with additional adjustments and nutritional supplements, his newly diagnosed mild-persistent asthma will be manageable without medication. His internist has prescribed medication and would like him to establish his personal best with a peak flow meter. How well do you think Joe will adhere to either treatment plan?

Drug Therapy Problems

Once you have identified therapy problems and formulated your TPL (refer to unit 5 for a discussion of the TPL), you will use these identified problems to develop pharmacotherapeutic and related health care goals for a patient. If there are multiple therapy problems, you may want to change only the most glaring things the first time that you see the patient. Making too many changes at one time may lead to:

- the patient experiencing discomfort with either your abilities or the abilities of the prescribing practitioner,
- difficulty interpreting unexpected outcomes,
- increased patient confusion about the care plan, and
- inability to distinguish which therapy is working, not working, or causing adverse reactions.

As with any patient, the goal of medication therapy for a patient with asthma is the provision of the lowest effective dose that is associated with minimal side effects. Corticosteroid therapy often raises fears in patients with asthma. Steroid abuse by athletes and the long-term Cushingoid effects of oral steroids have been reported widely by the press. It is often difficult for patients to distinguish between the available steroids and dosage forms. Pharmacotherapeutic goals common to asthma patients include:

- minimization of need for rescue $beta_2$-adrenergic agonist therapy and
- minimization of use of systemic corticosteroids.

Consider Scott Patrick, age 8. His mother has resisted the initiation of inhaled corticosteroids for Scott because of fears about steroid addiction and long-term side effects. Scott has had many exacerbations over the past year. On careful questioning, the pharmacist discovers Scott has had eight emergency room visits, and after each visit a short course of oral prednisone was prescribed. Scott's mother does not recognize the significance of these eight steroid bursts and the effects this type of exposure might have on Scott.

Jeremy Morgan's mother indicated that she also would prefer that Jeremy not take a corticosteroid. She has a friend who is taking corticosteroids following a renal transplant and is concerned that Jeremy will also experience some of the physical changes her friend is experiencing. Mrs. Morgan is also concerned about the connotation of steroid use and that, even if Jeremy's symptoms were under control and he could return to cross-country, he would be disqualified because of his use of steroids.

Patient-Related Factors

There is no single comprehensive description of an ambulatory care patient with asthma. Patients differ by age, educational background, and support structure. All these factors are important as you design pharmacotherapeutic and related health care goals for your patients.

Patients in different geographic areas have different needs. Patients with environmental triggers such as outdoor allergies may need to modify their activities to avoid hours and seasons with high pollen counts. Some areas of the country have higher pollen and spore counts than others. Moving from one area of the country to another can either worsen or improve symptoms in some patients with asthma. Crowded or unsanitary urban areas present problems for patients with sensitivity to cockroach allergen.

A patient's age is a significant consideration in the development of goals. In managing a pediatric patient with asthma, therapy is simplified on the one hand, because most pediatric patients have only one disease state to consider. It is complicated on the other hand by the inclusion of parents and their perception and capabilities into the development of goals. Several reasons exist for why parental reporting may be biased[2]:

- Parents may accept the current symptoms as normal.
- Parents might prefer their child not be on medication regularly, and may, therefore, under-report symptoms.
- Parents may present an edited version of their observations to you so that you don't make a qualitative decision about them or their child.
- Parents may not be aware of their child's actual activity level.

As discussed in unit 1, children should also be included in discussion about therapy or symptom reporting. Children have their own biases. A child's control of his or her symptoms will mean an expense of some time during the day, and the desire to manipulate this time may affect the child's reporting. It is wise to keep in mind that children tend to be slow in answering questions; often a parent will interrupt before the child has a chance to complete a thought.[2]

Goals for children need to include normal physiological growth and development as well as normal psychosocial development. Children with asthma are at risk for abnormal psychosocial development.[2] Pharmacotherapeutic and related health care goals for children with asthma must be designed to minimize the development of anxiety states, school absenteeism, peer-group ridicule, and social isolation.[2]

Pharmacotherapeutic and related health care goals for geriatric patients with asthma are complicated by the frequent coexistence of other diseases. The goals set by other health care providers for those diseases must be taken into consideration as the goals for asthma management are designed. Also, geriatric patients will often have caregivers who should be included in the goal setting for the patient. It would be difficult to insist that a patient receive medication four times a day when there is no caregiver to assist during two of those times and the patient is unable to administer the medications alone. In some instances, the same characteristics discussed for pediatric caregivers may also apply (e.g., perception of symptoms, caregiver control of medications, etc.).

Adult ambulatory patients with asthma have their own concerns that need to be addressed as pharmacotherapeutic and related health care goals are established. The ability to perform on the job, in classes, or at home are important considerations for these patients.

A patient's educational level is also important as you define pharmacotherapeutic and related health care goals for patients. Complicated medication regimens and monitoring procedures that stress the importance of following written instructions or require the patient to record information on charts necessitate that the patient is able to read and write at a sophisticated level. Functional health literacy cannot be assumed. Patients at two urban public hospitals were surveyed using a tool to evaluate functional health literacy.[3] Inadequate health literacy was found in 35.1% of English-speaking patients surveyed and 61.7% of Spanish-speaking patients. Color-coded action plans are available for patients (see unit 6); however, some reading is still required.

Quality of Life

Quality of life is a term that is used frequently in health care, and an assumption is made that the meaning is understood. For the purposes of this discussion, we will define quality of life as a patient's perception of the functional effects of his or her disease and its treatment. Quality of life is a personal assessment. It cannot be assessed by you as this would introduce your own biases into the assessment. Parents and caregivers may have their own interpretations of quality-of-life issues as the disease affects them and their ability to function at what they consider normal for them. Quality-of-life issues that frequently surface when patients with asthma are questioned include:

- sleeping through the night,
- maintaining a normal social life,
- participating in sports or exercise,
- attending school or work with minimal absences, and
- not needing to use medications in front of peers.

Quality of life can be measured in clinical studies but the instrument must be validated for both the disease and the age group being evaluated. General quality-of-life instruments may not provide enough information to health care providers that relates specifically to the issues that patients with asthma face daily. Quality-of-life instruments must be validated for specific populations and ethnic groups as well.

Most important in evaluating quality of life, be sure to ask patients what is important to them. Do not assume that you can guess; you might be wrong.

Consider Amy Gustafson, age 13. She had to quit the volleyball team, her mother reports, because of her asthma. Her mother insists that the ability to play on the volleyball team is extremely important to Amy and the rest of the family. The whole family is competitive, running in marathons and playing in recreational leagues of different sports. Volleyball has been the only sport that Amy has been able to play.

On questioning Amy alone about her goals for her health, without prompting her about the volleyball, she refers to not wanting to stand out among her peers. She suggests that by participating in volleyball, her need to use medications at the school nurse's office before practice was drawing attention to her disease. She does not describe treatment failure. Mother and daughter have the same issue, but very different assessments.

Ethical Issues

Unit 4 of this module covered many of the ethical issues that are important to consider when developing pharmacotherapeutic and related health care goals for ambulatory care patients with asthma. Issues such as use of medications or monitoring at school and work, environmental safety issues for children, and confidentiality are necessary considerations.

Jeremy Morgan's case provides an example of confidentiality concerns. He has confided to you that he has experimented with alcohol and tobacco. Although a goal of therapy for Jeremy will be to avoid use of these substances, enlisting the help of his parents must be his own decision and cannot be done by you without his permission.

The Role of Ambulatory Care Patients with Asthma in Determining Their Goals

As emphasized throughout this module, the patient must be considered an active participant, not only in carrying out a treatment plan, but also in design of the plan. The patient's readiness to accept this role will vary. Assessing the ability or willingness of a patient, parent, or caregiver to take on these responsibilities will aid in the success of the treatment plan. The patient's health belief and motivation as well as his or her quality-of-life assessment must be considered in the development of goals. All these factors influence the patient's ability and desire to carry out the treatment plan.

Health Beliefs

According to the Health Belief Model, patients conduct their own cost-benefit analysis with regard to treatments proposed by their health care provider.[4] Once established, these beliefs are difficult to alter. The Health Belief Model states that patients are most likely to adhere to treatment plans when:

- they perceive their illness to be significant and
- they believe the proposed treatment will be effective without adverse consequences (e.g., adverse effects of medications, financial sacrifice, or lifestyle change).

Patients listen to other patients with asthma talk about their therapy, read in the newspaper about the inadequacies of today's health care system, and read articles about the side effects of medications and the emergence of alternative therapies. This input frames the attitudes and beliefs of patients about therapies. Arguing with a belief is not always in a patient's best interest. You may need to alter your goals to accommodate patients' strong beliefs, as long as the alternatives are not harmful to patients and will ultimately facilitate positive outcomes. With time, you may be successful, in some circumstances, in providing patients with enough information to alter their health belief.

Motivation

In addition to the beliefs held by patients, it is their motivation or readiness for change that will enable them to achieve the goals that are set to be carried out. Another model exists to evaluate a patient's readiness to change. It is called the Transtheoretical or Stages-of-Change Model. The model describes five stages a patient can be at for any given behavior. These stages include:

- *Precontemplation*—a patient has no intention of changing behavior in the foreseeable future.
- *Contemplation*—a patient is aware that a problem exists and is seriously thinking about changing behavior in the next 6 months.
- *Preparation*—a patient intends to take action in the next month to change behavior.
- *Action*—a patient modifies his or her behavior for a period of time from 1 day to 6 months.
- *Maintenance*—a patient works to prevent relapse; a behavior change has been consistently maintained for at least 6 months.

You can ask questions about a particular goal to see where in these five stages a patient falls. An understanding of the stages will help you tailor goals and action plans to a patient's readiness to change. In this manner, you will provide the patient with incremental victory that might enable additional goals to be set.

Adherence

Once goals are established, you expect the patient to adhere to the pharmacotherapeutic plan that will facilitate achievement of those goals. The term *compliance* has been changed to *adherence* to remove the connotation that patients must simply obey a prescriber's orders.[5] Adherence implies that the goals and plan have been mutually agreed on. Working with a patient in a partnership and including communication with other members of the health care team in the treatment plan will facilitate adherence to a plan. Other factors that affect adherence include[6]:

- costs of treatment;
- methods of treatment delivery;
- complexity of the regimen;
- appearance, taste, and side effects of medications;
- communication between the patient and members of the health care team;
- effects of treatment on patient's quality of life; and
- the patient's perception of the effectiveness of treatment.

Keeping these factors in mind as you identify pharmacotherapeutic and related health care goals for your patients may affect the success of your interventions. Nonadherence to therapy is not intentional with most patients. In many cases of nonadherence, the goals of the plan are either not consistent with personal goals or are adversely affecting the patient in some manner.

Case Study

Let's return to the case of Jeremy Morgan (see unit 4, Appendix B, and unit 5, Appendix B). His completed goals are outlined in **Appendix A** at the end of this unit. He has been on inhaled corticosteroids for a year and was provided with a peak flow meter at the same time. Jeremy's mother assumes Jeremy is using his corticosteroid inhaler as prescribed; your refill records indicate otherwise. Jeremy has already told you that he does not use his peak flow meter. In trying to discover the regimen that Jeremy is following for his inhaled corticosteroids, you have the following conversation.

PHARMACIST:
"It's often difficult to remember to take medications exactly as the doctor prescribed them. How many times in a week do you think you forget to use your corticosteroid inhaler?"

JEREMY:
"Maybe two or three times."

PHARMACIST:
"Taking something four times a day is a lot to remember. Only missing a couple of times a week is super. What times of day do you usually use your corticosteroid inhaler?"

JEREMY:
"In the morning, at lunchtime, after school, and, uh, at bedtime."

PHARMACIST:
"Does the school nurse keep your inhaler at school?"

JEREMY:
"Yeah. And I feel foolish going down there."

PHARMACIST:
"I can imagine that might be very uncomfortable. Are those the doses you usually miss?"

JEREMY:
"Well, I actually don't do that one anymore."

PHARMACIST:
"Do you use your corticosteroid inhaler before you go to sleep?"

JEREMY:
"I skip that dose, too. Too many drugs at that time, I can't coordinate it."

Although the regimen described above is not clinically sound, Jeremy has designed his own regimen that meets his needs, and he is adherent to it. When asked how many times he forgets to take his medication, he only considers the doses in his own regimen when he refers to missed doses. In his case, one option would be to change the corticosteroid inhaler to one that can be used twice a day. Leukotriene receptor antagonists and long-acting $beta_2$-adrenergic agonists could also be considered. Any of these options will facilitate adherence, both to Jeremy's regimen and to the one his practitioner believes will provide the best health outcome.

On the APCP, we identified a problem list for Jeremy Morgan. Considering all the factors we have discussed, what pharmacotherapeutic and related health care goals have we identified for Jeremy? Let's review them and record them on the APCP.

- Minimize symptoms of disease; Jeremy's nighttime symptoms are particularly a problem for him.
- Optimize his medication use and find a regimen that will enable adherence.
- Protect the confidentiality of his experimentation with alcohol and tobacco while educating him about the risks associated with this behavior.
- Add peak flow monitoring to Jeremy's routine.
- Provide education to enable Jeremy to recognize symptoms and identify triggers.
- Discontinue therapy that is no longer providing a benefit (e.g., Echinacea).
- Add yearly influenza vaccine to Jeremy's care plan.
- Provide education to both Jeremy and his mother about corticosteroid use to minimize their misconceptions.

See **Appendix A** to see how this information has been recorded.

Realistic Treatment Outcomes for Ambulatory Care Patients with Asthma

One of the most important aspects of selecting a pharmacotherapeutic goal is choosing one that is achievable for the patient. The success or failure of interventions you suggest will have a direct impact on your future ability to have success with the patient. Patients must have realistic goals for the treatment of their disease. For most patients, asthma and asthma symptoms are lifelong considerations. Patients must understand that treatment goals can include preventing severe and frequent exacerbations but cannot be interpreted as curative.

There is a perception that asthma is a bothersome disease with some severe exacerbations but is not life threatening. This belief may be particularly prevalent among adolescent patients with asthma because, in general, they have feelings of immortality. In fact, asthma deaths do occur; **Table 1** lists the mortality rate by 10-year age groups per 100,000 population during the years 1979–1995. The mortality rate is increasing with time, not decreasing. This is a fact that many patients with asthma do not know.

Each ambulatory care setting is unique. Some practices are structured to allow more physical assessment and laboratory testing than is possible in other settings. In some practices, access to other health care practitioners and information that will facilitate goal setting and achievement is easier than in other sites. These limitations of ambulatory care practice must be considered when designing goals to ensure they are realistic.

The main goal of asthma treatment is to gain control of the disease. Treatment regimens offer a means of achieving this goal. Setting a treatment regimen for Jeremy Morgan that includes daily therapy in the school nurse's office sets the therapy plan up for failure right from the start. Jeremy has already indicated that this is an unacceptable alternative for him. This goal would be unrealistic.

Table 1. Mortality Rates

Year	Total	<1[a]	1–4	5–14	15–24	25–34	35–44	45–54	55–64	65–74	75–84	85+
1979	1.2	...	...[a]	0.1	0.2	0.3	0.6	1.2	2.3	4.5	6.6	8.6
1980	1.3	...	0.2	0.2	0.2	0.4	0.6	1.4	2.4	4.9	7.7	9.9
1981	1.3	...	...[a]	0.2	0.3	0.4	0.7	1.4	2.8	5.1	7.2	9.7
1982	1.4	...	0.2	0.2	0.4	0.4	0.6	1.5	2.6	4.9	7.2	9.6
1983	1.5	...	0.2	0.2	0.4	0.5	0.8	1.7	3.1	5.1	8.2	11.5
1984	1.5	...	...[a]	0.2	0.3	0.4	0.7	1.6	3.0	5.4	8.1	11.7
1985	1.6	...	0.1	0.3	0.4	0.4	0.7	1.7	3.4	5.6	8.8	12.4
1986	1.6	...	...[a]	0.3	0.4	0.5	0.8	1.6	3.1	5.7	9.2	12.8
1987	1.8	...	...[a]	0.3	0.5	0.5	1.0	1.9	3.3	6.2	9.3	14.5
1988	1.9	...	...[a]	0.3	0.4	0.5	1.0	1.8	3.6	6.2	10.3	14.9
1989	2.0	...	0.2	0.3	0.4	0.6	1.0	1.9	3.5	6.8	11.1	15.9
1990	1.9	...	0.2	0.3	0.4	0.5	0.9	2.0	3.5	6.2	10.7	16.9
1991	2.0	...	0.2	0.3	0.5	0.7	1.0	2.0	3.5	6.3	11.3	17.5
1992	1.9	...	0.2	0.2	0.5	0.5	0.9	1.8	3.3	6.3	10.4	18.7
1993	2.0	...	0.2	0.3	0.5	0.6	1.0	1.8	3.5	6.4	10.4	18.3
1994	2.1	...	0.2	0.3	0.6	0.7	1.0	2.0	3.7	6.5	10.6	18.3
1995	2.1	...	0.1	0.3	0.6	0.7	1.2	2.1	3.7	6.1	10.7	18.3

[a]Figures do not meet standard of reliability or precision (estimate based on <20 deaths).

Source: reference 7.

Likewise, trying to meet Jeremy's mother's goal of no continuous corticosteroid therapy for Jeremy may also be unrealistic.

Example Case

Realistic goals include recognition of the patient's ultimate goals. Consider the following case. Molly Cohen, age 11, has been coming to the asthma clinic since she was 4 years old. You are the pharmacist in this ambulatory clinic and have been seeing Molly since she was 7 years old. At each visit, you review Molly's inhaler technique and her understanding of her disease in addition to reviewing her medications. Lately, Molly has had three hospital admissions for her asthma; the last admission was to the ICU. Her pulmonologist is referring Molly back to you for therapy regimen adherence issues that she feels are responsible for Molly's current health change. The pulmonologist feels that the closer Molly gets to adolescence, the less adherent she is with her current regimen. However, something about the scenario the pulmonologist describes does not seem right. You know that Molly has always had a good attitude toward her disease and has always demonstrated an appropriate understanding of her disease, medications, and need for chronic treatment. In Molly's hospital record, you find mention of divorce proceedings from the inpatient social worker. When you see Molly, you confirm that she has a good understanding of the severity of her illness, the importance and functions of her medications, and the consequences of not taking the medications as prescribed. On questioning Molly casually about her home life, she becomes angry and quiet. Finally, Molly jokingly remarks that when she is in the hospital, her parents agree on something. When her mother joins the discussion, Molly answers no further questions and her mother appears frustrated with Molly, herself, and the disease. Establishing additional educational goals for Molly and her family might only set them back. Molly's understanding of her disease is allowing her to manipulate it to try to rectify home issues. Educational goals would, more than likely, be unrealistic at this point.

What goals would you establish for Molly? She will need a referral to a social worker to help her find support for her emotions about her parents' impending divorce. Helping Molly identify another health care provider who can aid her in finding a constructive way to deal with her anger will ultimately help her with her symptom control.

Practice Example

Let's return to the case of Mr. Kelley (see unit 4, Appendix C and D, and unit 5, Appendix C). Review the TPL and APCP that was created in unit 5. Consider Mr. Kelley's unique factors and issues and develop pharmacotherapeutic and related health care goals for him. Complete the third column of the APCP in **Appendix B**. When you are finished, compare your plan to the completed one in **Appendix C**. If you have any deficiencies you may want to review this unit, or the corresponding units in the *Core Module*.

Summary

All pharmaceutical care plans must have goals that direct therapy recommendations. These goals should address identified problems and meet each health care need. These goals must encompass the person as a whole. To do this, the goals must integrate disease characteristics, goals of other health care professionals, therapy problems, nondisease factors, and patient preferences. The goals must be realistic for each patient.

References

1. National Heart, Lung, and Blood Institute. Expert Panel Report 2: Guidelines for the Diagnosis and Management of Asthma. July 1997.
2. Pedersen S. What are the goals of treating pediatric asthma? *Pediatr Pulmonol Suppl* 1997;15:22–6.
3. Williams MV, Parker RM, Baker DW, et al. Inadequate functional health literacy among patients at two public hospitals. JAMA 1995;274:1677–82.
4. Bender B, Milgrom H, Rand C. Nonadherence in asthmatic patients: is there a solution to the problem? *Ann Allergy Asthma Immunol* 1997;79:177–86.
5. Milgrom H, Bender B. Nonadherence to asthma treatment and failure of therapy. *Curr Opin Pediatr* 1997;9:590–5.
6. Schmier JK, Leidy NK. The complexity of treatment adherence in adults with asthma: challenges and opportunities. *J Asthma* 1998;35:455–72.
7. American Lung Association (Epidemiology and Statistics Unit). Trends in Asthma Morbidity and Mortality. November 1998.

Self-Study Questions

Objective

Explain factors unique to ambulatory care patients with asthma that may influence decisions about pharmacotherapeutic and related health care goals, including:
- *disease characteristics of asthma,*
- *common goals of other health care professionals,*
- *common drug therapy problems,*
- *patient-related factors,*
- *quality-of-life issues, and*
- *ethical issues.*

1. Explain why disease characteristics are an important consideration when making decisions about pharmacotherapeutic and related health care goals for ambulatory care patients with asthma.

2. Explain why common goals of other health care professionals are an important consideration when making decisions about pharmacotherapeutic and related health care goals for ambulatory care patients with asthma.

3. Explain why quality-of-life issues are an important consideration when making decisions about pharmacotherapeutic and related health care goals for ambulatory care patients with asthma.

Objective

Explain the role of ambulatory care patients with asthma in determining their therapy goals.

4. Explain the role of ambulatory care patients in determining their therapy goals.

5. Explain why ambulatory care patients with asthma should have a role in determining their therapy goals.

6. Explain why a patient's health beliefs affect the patient's role in determining therapy goals.

Objective

Explain realistic limits of treatment outcomes for patients with asthma in the ambulatory care setting.

7. Explain realistic limits of treatment outcomes for ambulatory care patients with asthma.

8. Explain why the chronic nature of asthma is a realistic limit of treatment outcomes for an ambulatory care patient with asthma.

9. Explain why the ambulatory practice setting may be a realistic limit of treatment outcomes when caring for an ambulatory care patient with asthma.

Objective

Specify pharmacotherapeutic and related health care goals for an ambulatory care patient with asthma that integrate patient-specific data, disease-specific and medication-specific information, and ethical and quality-of-life considerations.

10. Refer to the case of Marie Cowling in unit 4, Appendixes E and F, and unit 5, Appendix E. Use the APCP at the end of this unit in **Appendix D** to record pharmacotherapeutic and related health care goals for this patient.

Self-Study Answers

1. An understanding of the course of asthma is important to the establishment of pharmacotherapeutic and related health care goals. The episodic nature of asthma will necessitate the establishment of immediate and long-term goals.

2. You must consider the goals established by other health care professionals when determining your goals to avoid conflicting messages, enable reinforcement of goals, and develop a comprehensive treatment plan that satisfies the whole team including the patient.

3. Quality-of-life issues are the perceptions the patient has about the functional effects of his or her disease and its treatments. These perceptions influence the patient's acceptance of the plan and the goals of therapy. These issues are unique to each patient and, therefore, must be elicited prior to setting goals for the patient's therapy.

4. Ambulatory care patients have an important role in determining their therapy goals. Their health beliefs and motivation must be considered.

5. Ambulatory care patients with asthma, as with any disease, have the primary responsibility of carrying out the therapy plan and achieving goals. They must be included in the development of these goals to facilitate their understanding and encourage acceptance of the responsibility for carrying out the plan.

6. Health beliefs are perceptions patients hold that influence their acceptance of a goal or therapy plan. Often these beliefs are difficult to change and present a significant barrier to successful implementation of a plan or achievement of a goal.

7. Realistic limits of treatment outcomes for ambulatory care patients with asthma include the limitations of the practice site, the chronic nature of the disease, and educational barriers (e.g., the lack of knowledge of the mortality associated with the disease).

8. The chronic nature of asthma limits the treatment goals to minimization of symptoms and exacerbations rather than curing the disease.

9. The ambulatory practice setting may have limited access to other health care professionals and information, but that should not limit the treatment goals that are achievable.

10. Compare your APCP with the completed one in **Appendix E**. If you have any deficiencies, you may want to review this unit, or the corresponding units in the *Core Module*.

Ambulatory Pharmacist's Care Plan

Patient: Jeremy Morgan   Pharmacist: Jennifer Loudon   Date: March 10, 1999

DATE IDENTIFIED	PROBLEM (TPL)	PHARMACOTHERAPEUTIC AND RELATED HEALTH CARE GOAL	RECOMMENDATIONS FOR THERAPY	MONITORING PARAMETER(S)	DESIRED ENDPOINT(S)	MONITORING FREQUENCY
3/99	overuse of Albuterol	minimize symptoms, optimize therapeutic regimen				
	intermittent refill record Azmacort	optimize education & medication administration				
	cigarette & alcohol use	protect confidentiality while educating about risks				
	self-monitoring not done	Add peak flow monitoring				
	poor symptom recognition	Educate about symptoms				
	Echinacea use for prolonged time	Discontinue Echinacea				
	Influenza vaccine: Not vaccinated	Vaccinate yearly				
	Misconceptions about corticosteroids	Provide Education				

© 2000, American Society of Health-System Pharmacists, Inc. All rights reserved.

Ambulatory Pharmacist's Care Plan

Patient __Mike Kelley__ Pharmacist __Bob Jones__ Date __5/5/99__

DATE IDENTIFIED	PROBLEM (TPL)	PHARMACOTHERAPEUTIC AND RELATED HEALTH CARE GOAL	RECOMMENDATIONS FOR THERAPY	MONITORING PARAMETER(S)	DESIRED ENDPOINT(S)	MONITORING FREQUENCY
5/5/99	Drug-disease interaction (ibuprofen)					
	No self-monitoring					
	Needs baseline education					
6/12/99	Continued symptoms					
	Nonadherence to treatment plan					

© 2000, American Society of Health-System Pharmacists, Inc. All rights reserved.

Ambulatory Pharmacist's Care Plan

Patient **Mike Kelley** Pharmacist **Bob Jones** Date **5/5/99**

DATE IDENTIFIED	PROBLEM (TPL)	PHARMACOTHERAPEUTIC AND RELATED HEALTH CARE GOAL	RECOMMENDATIONS FOR THERAPY	MONITORING PARAMETER(S)	DESIRED ENDPOINT(S)	MONITORING FREQUENCY
5/5/99	Drug-disease interaction (ibuprofen)	No interaction				
	No self-monitoring	Daily PEF monitoring				
	Needs baseline education	Knowledge of disease management				
6/12/99	Continued symptoms	No symptoms				
	Nonadherence to treatment plan	Adherence				

© 2000, American Society of Health-System Pharmacists, Inc. All rights reserved.

Ambulatory Pharmacist's Care Plan

Patient __Marie Cowling__ Pharmacist __John Bellows__ Date __July 8, 1999__

DATE IDENTIFIED	PROBLEM (TPL)	PHARMACOTHERAPEUTIC AND RELATED HEALTH CARE GOAL	RECOMMENDATIONS FOR THERAPY	MONITORING PARAMETER(S)	DESIRED ENDPOINT(S)	MONITORING FREQUENCY
7/8/99	Overuse of Beta-adrenergic agonist					
→	No local health care provider					
→	No PEF monitoring					
→	Possible drug-disease interaction					
→	improved disease control					
→	Arthritis					

© 2000, American Society of Health-System Pharmacists, Inc. All rights reserved.

Ambulatory Pharmacist's Care Plan

Patient __Marie Cowling__   Pharmacist __John Bellows__   Date __July 8, 1999__

DATE IDENTIFIED	PROBLEM (TPL)	PHARMACOTHERAPEUTIC AND RELATED HEALTH CARE GOAL	RECOMMENDATIONS FOR THERAPY	MONITORING PARAMETER(S)	DESIRED ENDPOINT(S)	MONITORING FREQUENCY
	Overuse of Beta-adrenergic agonist	Use Beta-adrenergic agonist appropriately & have good disease control				
	No local health care provider	Establish relationship with local physician				
	No PEF monitoring	PEF monitoring				
	Possible drug-disease interaction	No drug-disease interaction				
	improved disease control	Asthma control				
	Arthritis	control of arthritis symptoms				

© 2000, American Society of Health-System Pharmacists, Inc. All rights reserved.

Ambulatory Pharmacist's Care Plan

Patient _Mary Franklin_   Pharmacist _Cheryl Marks_   Date _9/20/99_

DATE IDENTIFIED	PROBLEM (TPL)	PHARMACOTHERAPEUTIC AND RELATED HEALTH CARE GOAL	RECOMMENDATIONS FOR THERAPY	MONITORING PARAMETER(S)	DESIRED ENDPOINT(S)	MONITORING FREQUENCY
9/20/99	Overuse of Beta-adrenergic Agonist					
	No local provider					
	No PEF monitoring					
	Baseline Education					
	Asthma poorly controlled					

© 2000, American Society of Health-System Pharmacists, Inc. All rights reserved.

Designing a Therapy Regimen for Patients with Asthma

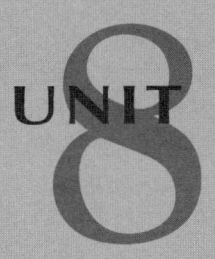
UNIT 8

Unit Objectives	198
Unit Organization	198
Factors That Influence the Design of a Therapy Regimen	198
Patient-Related Concerns	198
Treatment Guidelines	199
Designing and Selecting Patient-Specific Education	201
Asthma Overview	203
Role of Medications	203
Skills	203
Example Case	203
Environmental Control Measures	203
Rescue Medications: Action Plan	203
Case Study	206
Educational Process	207
Potential Sources of Patient-Specific Education	208
Designing a Therapy Regimen	208
Case Study	213
Practice Example	213
Summary	214
References	214
Self-Study Questions	215
Self-Study Answers	217
Appendixes	219

In the previous unit, you learned how to identify pharmacotherapeutic and related health care goals. In this unit you will learn the next phase: how to design a therapy regimen based on these goals and your patient's health care needs. A therapy regimen is basically a listing of recommendations to achieve the pharmacotherapeutic and related health care goals you have established for a patient. These recommendations will be documented on the ambulatory care pharmacist's care plan (APCP).

The process used to design the therapy regimen can be found in unit 14 (Figure 1) of the *Core Module*. You will want to review the steps in this process before reading further. After you have identified pharmacotherapeutic and related health care goals, you must prioritize them and decide which goals to address first. You must then develop recommendations to achieve these goals. These recommendations make up your therapy regimen, which may be simple or complex. As you design the therapy regimen for a patient with asthma, you need to consider patient- and medication-related factors, nonpatient factors, and existing treatment guidelines.

Unit Objectives

After you successfully complete this unit, you will be able to:
- explain how patient-related concerns unique to ambulatory care patients with asthma may influence the design of their therapy regimens;
- explain the use of treatment guidelines in the design of therapy regimens for ambulatory care patients with asthma;
- explain education needs unique to ambulatory care patients with asthma;
- explain factors unique to ambulatory care patients with asthma that affect the approaches used for education;
- explain what is unique about the role of preventive education in patient-specific education for ambulatory care patients with asthma;
- state potential education resources used to meet an ambulatory asthma patient's educational needs so the patient may successfully participate in the pharmacist's care plan; and
- design a therapy regimen, including patient-specific education, that meets the pharmacotherapeutic and related health care goals established for an ambulatory care patient with asthma, integrates patient-specific disease and drug information as well as ethical and quality-of-life issues, and considers pharmacoeconomic principles.

Unit Organization

To begin, this unit describes factors that influence design of the therapy regimen for ambulatory care patients with asthma. Next, we discuss the process of designing and selecting patient-specific education for ambulatory care patients with asthma. Finally, we use a case study to illustrate the process of designing a therapy regimen for an ambulatory care patient with asthma.

Factors That Influence the Design of a Therapy Regimen

Patient-Related Concerns

Throughout the *Core Module* and this module, we have discussed factors that may be present in a patient's life that will influence your design of a therapy regimen. In this section, we highlight several important patient factors to consider in the treatment of a patient with asthma. Underlying these patient-related factors is the patient's perception of asthma and the risk for morbidity and mortality as a result of the disease. If a patient does not believe that asthma is a serious, fatal disease, he or she will be less likely to actively participate in the care plan and adhere to recommendations. If a perception of the seriousness of asthma is present, educational efforts designed to help the patient understand asthma and the potential consequences of poorly controlled disease will be a priority. Patient satisfaction with asthma care will also be factored into a patient's decision to comply with therapy. **Table 1** lists several questions you should consider asking a patient. A patient's response to these questions should be incorporated into your treatment decisions and pharmacotherapeutic plan.

A patient's age and physical coordination must be considered in the design of any medication regimen. Children need a parent or caregiver to administer and keep track of their medications and

> **Table 1. Monitoring Patient Satisfaction**
>
> - How satisfied are you with your asthma care?
> - How can we improve your asthma care?
> - Have the costs of your asthma treatment interfered with your ability to get asthma care?
> - Has anything prevented you from getting the treatment you need for your asthma from me or anyone else?
> - What problems have you had following your daily self-management plan? Your action plan?
> - What questions have you had about your asthma daily self-management plan and action plan?

Source: reference 1.

any monitoring. The child's caregiver needs to be a reliable person who will be able to assist the child with disease management. Caregiver issues hold true for any patient, including physically disabled and geriatric patients. Because young children lack the physical coordination necessary to activate an inhaler, they will need to use spacer devices or nebulizers with inhaled medications. Beyond the use in pediatrics, spacers may also be useful:
- with inhaled corticosteroids to decrease systemic exposure,
- for geriatric patients, and
- for a patient having difficulty coordinating actuation.

As discussed in earlier units, children and adolescent patients need medication regimens that upset their school schedules least. The majority of school systems in the United States do not allow children to carry inhalers. In many states, legislation is being presented to alter this restriction. In most states, a school nurse or someone in the school office is required to keep medications; students must then ask permission to use their inhaler. It is obvious this can be prohibitive to patients with asthma. The need to ask someone else to use a medication will decrease adherence and serve to single a patient out as different. The use of smaller, palm-size inhalers (rotahalers) have been prescribed in some cases, so that children can keep them and use them more discreetly. **Table 2** lists aerosol delivery devices, including dry powder inhalers (rotahalers). In addition to the relevance of control of medications to therapy adherence, remember that many patients with asthma, adolescents in particular, rebel against the disease and purposefully omit medications and treatment recommendations.

As patients age, their health becomes more complicated. The presence of more than one disease complicates asthma management. For example, patients with arthritis or loss of strength may have difficulty actuating inhaler devices. Elderly patients typically take several medications. Multiple medications complicate medication regimens, present drug interaction challenges, and increase the chance of adverse effects. You will need to consider all of these factors as you work with your patient to develop a pharmacotherapeutic plan.

Environmental factors are a key consideration in the design of a therapy regimen. Patients who are sensitive to inhalant allergens need to be educated on the recognition and avoidance of these triggers. In some situations (e.g., work), avoidance may not be feasible and prophylactic strategies will need to be developed. This can include the prophylactic use of inhaled corticosteroids, short-acting $beta_2$-adrenergic agonists prior to exposure or as rescue, and immunotherapy where appropriate. Environmental tobacco smoke and pollution can trigger airway inflammation. House-dust mites, pet dander, and fungi are other common sources of environmental exposure, especially in pediatric asthma patients; household precautions need to be enforced. You need to have resources available to help patients understand how to make their home environment appropriate for a patient with asthma. The Expert Panel Report 2 contains a section on environmental control that will be helpful. A chart outlining environmental control measures can be found in **Table 3**. Also consider using your local American Lung Association branch for educational resources. Patients can be referred to numerous educational sources and Internet sites for further information. A list of resources can be found in **Table 4**.

Treatment Guidelines

In addition to the factors we have discussed and those in the *Core Module* unit 14, Figure 1, existing treatment guidelines influence the design of a therapy regimen. Guidelines are an important tool in patient care; however, they must be interpreted and applied with consideration of

Table 2. Aerosol Delivery Devices

Device/Drugs	Population	Optimal Technique	Therapeutic Issues
Metered-dose inhaler (MDI) • Beta$_2$-adrenergic agonists • Corticosteroids • Cromolyn sodium and nedocromil • Anticholinergics	>5 years	Actuation during a slow (30 L/min or 3–5 sec) deep inhalation, followed by 10-sec breath-holding. Under laboratory conditions, open-mouth technique (holding MDI 2 in. away from open mouth) enhances delivery to the lung. However, it has not consistently been shown to enhance clinical benefit compared to closed-mouth technique (closing lips around MDI mouthpiece).	Slow inhalation may be difficult. Difficulty with coordination of actuation and inhalation, particularly in young children and elderly. Patients may incorrectly stop inhalation at actuation. Deposition of 80% of actuated dose in oropharynx. Mouth washing is effective in reducing systemic absorption.
Breath-actuated MDI • Beta$_2$-adrenergic agonists	>5 years	Slow (30 L/min or 3–5 sec) inhalation followed by 10-sec breath-holding.	Indicated for patients unable to coordinate inhalation and actuation. May be particularly useful in elderly. Slow inhalation may be difficult and patients may incorrectly stop inhalation at actuation. Requires more rapid inspiration to activate than is optimal for deposition. Cannot be used with currently available spacer/holding chamber devices.
Dry powder inhaler (DPI) • Beta$_2$-adrenergic agonists • Corticosteroids		Rapid (60 L/min or 1–2 sec), deep inhalation. Minimally effective inspiratory flow is device dependent.	Dose lost if patient exhales through device. Delivery may be ≥MDI depending on device and technique. Can be used in children 4 years old, but effects are more consistent with children >5. Most appear to have similar delivery efficiency as MDI either with or without spacer/holding chamber, but some may have delivery >MDI. Mouth washing is effective in reducing systemic absorption.
Spacer/holding chamber	>4 years ≤4 years with face mask	Slow (30 L/min or 3–5 sec) inhalation or tidal breathing immediately following actuation. Actuation only once into spacer/holding chamber per inhalation. If face mask is used, allow 3–5 inhalations per actuation.	Easier to use than MDI alone. With a face mask, enables MDI to be used with small children. Simple tubes do not obviate coordinating actuation and inhalation. Bulky. Output may be reduced in some devices after cleaning. The larger volume spacers/holding chambers (>600 cc) may increase lung delivery over MDI alone in patients with poor MDI technique. The effect of a spacer/holding chamber on output from an MDI is dependent on both MDI and spacer type; thus, data from one combination should not be extrapolated to all others. Spacers/holding chambers decrease oropharyngeal deposition and will reduce potential system absorption of inhaled corticosteroid preparations that have higher oral bioavailability. Spacers/holding chambers are recommended for all patients on medium-to-high doses of inhaled corticosteroids. May be as effective as nebulizer in delivering high doses of beta$_2$-adrenergic agonists during severe exacerbations.

Table 2. Aerosol Delivery Devices (cont.)

Device/Drugs	Population	Optimal Technique	Therapeutic Issues
Nebulizer • Beta$_2$-adrenergic agonists • Cromolyn • Anticholinergics • Corticosteroids	≤2 years; patients of any age who cannot use MDI with spacer/holding chamber or spacer and face mask (e.g., during exacerbation).	Slow tidal breathing with occasional deep breaths. Tightly fitting face mask for those unable to use mouthpiece.	Less dependent on patient coordination or cooperation. Delivery method of choice for cromolyn in children and for high-dose beta$_2$-adrenergic agonists and anticholinergics in moderate-to-severe exacerbations in all patients. Expensive; time consuming; bulky; output is device dependent; significant internebulizer and intranebulizer output variances.

Source: reference 1.

regional and patient-specific circumstances. The Expert Panel Report 2 guidelines are national clinical practice guidelines available from the National Institutes of Health: National Heart, Lung, and Blood Institute.[1] These guidelines, finalized in July 1997, are an update to the original guidelines from 1991 and are available from the National Heart, Lung, and Blood Institute or can be downloaded from the Internet (www.nhlbi.nih.gov/guidelines/asthma/asthgdln.htm). The appropriate use of guidelines requires you to be aware of how current they are in view of possible advances in asthma management. The guidelines need to be adapted to individual patients based on their needs and circumstances. Many health care organizations have adapted these national guidelines to their own organization, forming more specific guidelines. Specific guidelines may suggest medications based on formulary choices or pharmacoeconomic factors. Remember to consider these specific guidelines—usually used by hospitals, managed care companies, insurers, and physician groups—when appropriate.

Designing and Selecting Patient-Specific Education

Asthma education is a significant part of asthma management. The majority of asthma management is provided by the patient. Self-management is the key to controlling asthma exacerbations. Understanding the disease will enable the patient to manage symptoms and prevent exacerbations. The goals of patient-specific education are to prevent problems from occurring and to solve problems if they occur. Preventing problems can be accomplished through proactive education and provision of a patient treatment and action plan. Proactive education teaches patients what they need to know to avoid problems with their medications, triggers, and exacerbations. For example, a well-educated patient with asthma knows what to do at the onset of an exacerbation to avoid worsening of the airway obstruction.

The Expert Panel Report 2 calls for a partnership with the patient in asthma care. The panel's guidelines devote a section to educating and acting as a partner with an asthma patient. Patient education should begin with the diagnosis of asthma and be intertwined with every aspect of asthma care. Asthma education is not the responsibility of a single health care team member, but rather a responsibility of all health care team members. Patients and their primary health care provider will jointly decide on treatment goals and an action plan. It is the role of the other health care team members to reinforce the plan and goals and expand on them as necessary. The goal is to have everyone advocating a single plan for the patient. Education should include:

- asthma overview: basic facts, stress and psychosocial adjustment, family involvement and social support, and exercise and activity;

Table 3. Summary of Control Measures for Environmental Factors That Can Make Asthma Worse

Allergens:

Reduce or eliminate exposure to the allergen(s) the patient is sensitive to, including:

- **Animal dander**: Remove animal from house or, at a minimum, keep animal out of patient's bedroom and seal or cover with a filter air ducts that lead to bedroom.
- **House-dust mites**:
  - *Essential*: Encase mattress in an allergen-impermeable cover; encase pillow in an allergen-impermeable cover or wash it weekly; wash sheets and blankets on the patient's bed in hot water weekly (water temperature of ≥130°F is necessary for killing mites).
  - *Desirable*: Reduce indoor humidity to <50%; remove carpets from the bedroom; avoid sleeping or lying on upholstered furniture; remove carpets that are laid on concrete.
- **Cockroaches**: Use poison bait or traps to control. Do not leave food or garbage exposed.
- **Pollens (from trees, grass, or weeds) and outdoor molds**: To avoid exposure, adults should stay indoors with windows closed during the season in which they have problems with outdoor allergens, especially during the afternoon.
- **Indoor mold**: Fix all leaks and eliminate water sources associated with mold growth; clean moldy surfaces. Consider reducing indoor humidity to <50%.

Tobacco Smoke:

Advise patients and others in the home who smoke to stop smoking or to smoke outside the home. Discuss ways to reduce exposure to other sources of tobacco smoke, such as from day care providers and the workplace.

Indoor/Outdoor Pollutants and Irritants:

Discuss ways to reduce exposures to the following:
- Wood-burning stoves or fireplaces
- Unvented stoves or heaters
- Other irritants (e.g., perfumes, cleaning agents, and sprays)

Source: reference 1.

Table 4. Educational Resources

- American Lung Association (1-800-LUNG-USA; www.lungusa.org); validated educational programs ("Open Airways at School"); other educational pieces; multi-language
- Asthma and Allergy Foundation of America (1-800-7-ASTHMA/www.aafa.org); validated educational programs ("Asthma Training Care for Kids" and "You Can Control Asthma"); other educational pieces; multi-language
- National Technical Information Service (1-703-487-4650); validated educational programs ("Air Power," "Air Wise," "Living with Asthma," and "Open Airways"); other educational pieces; multi-language
- National Asthma Education and Prevention Program (1-301-251-1222/www.nhlbi.nih.gov/nhlbi/nhlbi.htm); validated educational program; other educational materials; multi-language
- Allergy and Asthma Network/Mothers of Asthmatics, Inc. (1-800-878-4403/www.aanma.com); educational resources
- American Academy of Allergy, Asthma, and Immunology (1-800-822-ASTHMA/www.aaaai.org); educational resources
- American College of Allergy, Asthma, and Immunology (1-800-842-7777/www.allergy.mcg.edu); educational programs
- National Jewish Medical and Research Center (1-800-222-LUNG/www.njc.org); educational programs
- American Association for Respiratory Care (1-972-243-2272)
- Healthy Kids: The Key to the Basics (1-617-965-9637)

Additional educational resources may be obtained from pharmaceutical manufacturers. Many of the manufacturers have Web sites that offer educational programs and information for patients. Review all information on the manufacturer Web site before you suggest a patient use these resources. In addition, remember that as the market changes, educational pieces available on a specific drug on a manufacturer Web site may be replaced by the resources to support another product.

Source: reference 1.

- medications and their role;
- skills: inhaler technique (spacer/holding chamber use) and self-monitoring (use of peak flow meter);
- environmental control measures;
- rescue medication action plan: (which should include written daily self-management plan and action plan); and
- use of health care systems and community resources.

Providing a detailed education plan for a patient with asthma is beyond the scope of this document. Several excellent resources for patient education about asthma are available. Educational resources for patient education materials can be found later in this unit. The following discussion highlights important components of the education.

Asthma Overview

You need to make sure the patient understands asthma and its effect on the airways. It is helpful to teach patients the difference between normal airways and those of a patient with asthma. Help patients understand what happens to the airways in an asthma attack. Providing patients with a basic knowledge of asthma will help them understand their medications and the role of each medication in the management of their disease.

Role of Medications

You need to teach the patient about the overall goal of reducing airway inflammation with anti-inflammatory agents as well as clarify for the patient the role of anti-inflammatory agents compared to short-acting, quick-onset bronchodilators. Patients need to understand which medication to use for acute symptoms. The need for continued use of prophylactic or long-term control medications, such as anti-inflammatory agents, even when the patient is feeling fine, will need to be emphasized. Side effects and possible drug interactions should also be included in this discussion.

Skills

Medication skills, including inhaler technique and the correct use of a spacer/holding chamber, need to be reviewed at each patient visit. Inappropriate inhaler technique can lead to reduced medication efficacy. A handout outlining correct inhaler technique can be found in **Figure 1**. Correct use of peak flow meters and monitoring of symptoms should also be continually reinforced.

Symptom monitoring and signs of distress need to be continually reinforced. Patients should be encouraged to keep a daily symptom diary and document rescue medications or stepped-up therapy. A sample diary can be found in **Figure 2**. As discussed throughout this module, some patients learn to live with their symptoms and fail to recognize subtle signs of deterioration. Nighttime cough, increased need for rescue medications, and inability to participate in sports are often seen as normal for asthma patients but are really signs of poorly controlled disease.

Example Case

The need to reinforce a patient's monitoring technique can be observed in the following example. Julie Jones is a 10-year-old patient with asthma. She presented to the asthma clinic and spoke with the pharmacist about discontinuing her inhaled corticosteroid. She felt she no longer needed long-term anti-inflammatory agents because her disease had gotten much better. She was basing her disease improvement on peak flow readings that were above her predicted values for her height. However, on exam she was noted to have mild wheezing. The pharmacist then asked her to demonstrate use of her peak flow meter. During the demonstration, the pharmacist noted she was using her tongue to force air through the device. This caused falsely elevated peak flow readings. On checking her peak flow with proper technique she was in her yellow zone.

Environmental Control Measures

Patients need to understand their triggers and how to avoid environmental exposures. Patients need to understand what steps should be taken when an exposure triggers an asthma attack.

Rescue Medications: Action Plan

All patients should have a written, daily self-management plan that outlines their treatment goals and the role of each medication. In addition to this daily plan, a written action plan should be developed that outlines action steps in the event of an asthma exacerbation. This is especially important in patients with moderate-to-severe persistent asthma. This plan should provide an outline of medications adjustments the patient can implement at home in response to symptoms

Steps for using your inhaler

1. Remove the cap and hold inhaler upright.
2. Shake the inhaler.
3. Tilt your head back slightly and breathe out slowly.
4. Position the inhaler in one of the following ways (A or B is optimal, but C is acceptable for those who have difficulty with A or B. C is required for breath-activated inhalers):

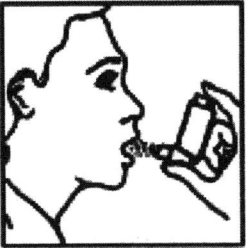 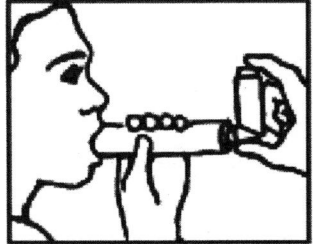 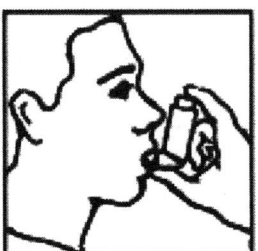 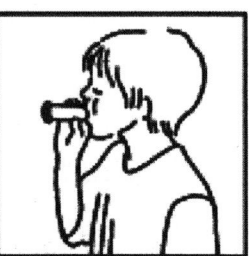

A. Open mouth with inhaler 1–2 inches away.

B. Use spacer/holding chamber (that is recommended especially for young children and for people using corticosteroids).

C. In the mouth. Do not use for corticosteroids.

D. *NOTE*: Inhaled dry powder capsules require a different inhalation technique. To use a dry powder inhaler, it is important to close the mouth tightly around the mouthpiece of the inhaler and to inhale.

5. Press down on the inhaler to release medication as you start to breathe in slowly.
6. Breathe in slowly (3–5 secs).
7. Hold your breath for 10 secs to allow the medicine to reach deeply into your lungs.
8. Repeat puff as directed. Waiting 1 min between puffs may permit second puff to penetrate your lungs better.
9. Spacers/holding chambers are useful for all patients. They are particularly recommended for young children and older adults and for use with inhaled corticosteroids.

Avoid common inhaler mistakes. Follow these inhaler tips:
- Breathe out before pressing your inhaler.
- Inhale slowly.
- Breathe in through your mouth, not your nose.
- Press down on your inhaler at the start of inhalation (or within the first second of inhalation).
- Keep inhaling as you press down on inhaler.
- Press your inhaler only once while you are inhaling (one breath for each puff).
- Make sure you breathe in evenly and deeply.

NOTE: Other inhalers are becoming available in addition to those illustrated above. Different types of inhalers may require different techniques.

Figure 1. Steps for using your inhaler
Source: reference 1.

Patient Self-assessment Diary

Date	Wheeze	Cough	Activity	Sleep	Quick Relief: Beta₂–Agonist	Cromolyn/Nedocromil	Inhaled Steroids	Other – Inhaled	Oral Steroids	Theophylline	Peak Flow			Comments
											AM	PM	Other Times	

Wheeze	None	= 0	Some	= 1	Medium	= 2	Severe = 3
Cough	None	= 0	Occasional	= 1	Frequent	= 2	Continuous = 3
Activity	Normal	= 0	Can run short distance or climb 3 flights of stairs	= 1	Can walk only	= 2	Missed school or work or stayed indoors = 3
Sleep	Fine	= 0	Slept well, slight wheeze or cough	= 1	Awake 2-3 times, wheeze or cough	= 2	Bad night, awake most of the time = 3

This diary is provided as an example for clinicians.

Figure 2. Patient self-assessment: example of patient diary
Source: reference 1.

and peak flow measurements. The plan should also indicate at which peak flow reading and group of symptoms the patient should contact the doctor or emergency room. Use of the health care system and community resources can be introduced with the action plan. Patients should be taught to self-manage their disease and control symptoms to reduce the need for emergency resources.

Case Study

Let's return to the case of Jeremy Morgan. What educational needs should be addressed with Jeremy? Jeremy has had asthma for years, and it has been fairly well controlled. As he enters his adolescent years, his exacerbations are becoming more frequent. He is unhappy having asthma and would like to forget he has a disease. His mother is caught in a transition period with Jeremy and his emerging independence. Educational efforts need to include both Jeremy and his mother. Even though asthma is not new to Jeremy, he needs basic asthma education that explains what happens to his airways during an exacerbation. Education needs to be directed at getting Jeremy to understand the potential seriousness of asthma when not adequately controlled. Jeremy needs reinforcement in recognition of symptoms and triggers. These are the most immediate needs that should be addressed. If Jeremy isn't able to grasp the seriousness of asthma, his willingness to adhere with a given treatment plan diminishes greatly. During the first session, the role of Jeremy's medications and his inhaler technique should also be addressed. Educational points that can be initiated at future sessions include:

- continued education about the seriousness of asthma;
- continued medication counseling;
- skills education (e.g., peak flow, spacer, and symptoms recognition);
- environmental control and recognition of triggers;
- daily self-management and action plan awareness; and
- use of health care systems and community resources.

Because Jeremy has a significant need for asthma education, you should schedule him for regular visits (about every 2 weeks) for the first couple of sessions. You should then see him every month or two to reinforce education. You should have him come and see you after any medication changes, physician visits, and exacerbations.

Let's see how Jeremy's pharmacist handles these issues in the following dialogue. Remember that this conversation between Jeremy and the pharmacist is confidential.

PHARMACIST:
"Jeremy, I've asked you a lot of questions today about your asthma and your life in general. I understand how difficult it is to be a teenager, especially with peer pressure. Having asthma means you need to be extra careful about some of the things you do. If we all work together, we will be able to help you learn to control your symptoms and reduce asthma attacks. I know you don't want to be lectured; you get enough of that everywhere else in your life. I need you to understand, however, how serious asthma can be."

JEREMY:
"I know, I've heard it all before. But you know, I could walk outside and get killed by a car right now. So what is the point? Why should I have to take all of the medications? It just makes me look even more like an outsider than I already do. I've never really heard of anyone dying from asthma, anyhow."

PHARMACIST:
"It's hard to imagine someone as young as yourself dying. I remember being your age and feeling like nothing in the world could hurt me. But the truth is asthma deaths do happen, and the incidence of people dying from asthma is increasing. Let me tell you about a former patient of mine. She was a 16-year-old girl who had asthma since she was little, much like you. When she got into high school, she rebelled against her parents, the doctors, everyone. She quit taking her medications and socialized in an atmosphere of out-of-control tobacco and alcohol use. She would end up in the emergency room at least once a month with an asthma exacerbation. Each time she came in she said she would start taking her medications at home and avoid environmental triggers, but this resolve to change her behavior never lasted. Somehow, no one was ever able to get through to her. The day after her last emergency room visit, she died at a friend's house. There was a big party and everyone was smoking. She couldn't breathe and her friends

didn't realize she was in trouble until it was too late. She did not differ significantly from other asthma patients or from other high school students in general. Deaths from asthma are unfortunate chiefly because they don't have to happen. You have the ability to control asthma instead of letting it control you. But you must take responsibility for controlling it. No one can do that for you. Just like no one could do it for that 16-year-old girl."

JEREMY:
"Wow, did that really happen or are you trying to scare me?"

PHARMACIST:
"It really happened, Jeremy, and I don't want you to end up the same way. I know how much you like computers, why don't you go on the Internet and check out the American Lung Association's Web site. The site gives you all sorts of numbers and information about asthma that you can check out for yourself. You can try going there when you get home; the Web site is www.lungusa.org. I know we've talked for a long time today, but I'd like to go over your medications quickly and the treatment plan you have from Dr. Lefton. We need to make sure you understand why each medication is used and what to do if your symptoms get worse. We can do this pretty quickly today and then sit down and talk again after you see Dr. Lefton to see how you are doing and talk about any changes in your medications. How does that sound?"

JEREMY:
"I know about all of my medicines, but we can go over them again."

Through the discussion about Jeremy's medications, the pharmacist identified that Jeremy and his mother really didn't have a clear understanding of the role of each medication. The pharmacist noted on her treatment plan that reinforcement of medications would need to continue. Jeremy demonstrated inhaler technique during his exacerbation. The pharmacist noted that he was using the inhaler properly.

The pharmacist provided Jeremy and his mother with written educational material about asthma from the American Lung Association. The pharmacist also provided Jeremy and his mother with the names of other places they could contact for information about asthma.

Educational Process

Unit 16 of the *Core Module* includes an overview of the educational process. You may want to refer to that unit to refresh your memory. We have already defined the content that is important in asthma education. You may need to modify the content based on a patient's particular needs. You will also need to break the education up into manageable pieces so that the patient and family are not overwhelmed. You can also consider conducting group classes about asthma management and open them up to your patients, families, friends, and school personnel. Educating school personnel about asthma and its management can help patients in the overall management of their disease.[3] Topics that should be covered in a group class could include:

- general overview of asthma and treatment options,
- new medications and developments in asthma management,
- educational resources for patients with asthma,
- question-and-answer session, and
- group dialogue to discuss personal solutions and problems facing asthma patients daily.

There are several patient factors that must be considered as you enter into the educational process with patients. These factors were discussed in unit 16 of the *Core Module* and include:

- level of patient education,
- cognitive ability,
- literacy,
- language comprehension,
- vision,
- hearing,
- physical limitations, and
- age.

In addition to these factors, patients (like the rest of us) have different learning styles. Some patients may prefer reading about how to perform a skill; others may learn better by example. The incorporation of visual materials, numerical presentations (the use of numbers to make a point; e.g., 1 in 5 patients experience a symptom or adverse effect), graphic directions, and demonstration will be necessary in the educational process. Inhaler and peak flow meter technique are best taught through demonstration and graphic directions. Encourage patients to use the Internet to review the list of Web sites listed in

Table 4 that address asthma. This can promote active learning and self-study by the patient. You need to caution your patients to decide if a source of information taken from the Internet is reliable. For example, information received from a chat room or advocacy group may not be medically valid. Encourage your patients to come to you for help deciding if information is medically sound. Other teaching strategies you may want to incorporate into your patient sessions are:
- lectures (large groups),
- discussions (good for support groups and informal settings),
- demonstrations,
- print materials,
- audiovisual presentations,
- role-playing,
- games,
- computer simulations, and
- case reviews.

Role-playing can be used to help teach patients how to tell their peers about asthma, deal with peer pressure, and even describe how an asthma exacerbation feels. Role-playing gives the patient an opportunity to act out a scenario before it actually happens. Computer simulations can be useful for helping patients learn how to self-manage their disease. Providing patients with potential scenarios and symptoms can help them learn what actions should be taken based on the presenting symptoms. Creative use of teaching strategies helps patients learn to effectively take control of their disease.

Keep in mind as you develop and provide education for your patients that prevention of exacerbations needs to be a key factor in your discussions. Patient education must reinforce that asthma is variable in nature and that prevention of exacerbations should be at the center of all treatment regimens.

Regardless of the educational materials you select, be sure to refer to the checklist for evaluating audio, written, and audiovisual educational materials in the *Core Module*, unit 16, Figure 1. This will help you match educational materials to your patients' needs.

Potential Sources of Patient-Specific Education

Many sources of asthma education materials are available. A list of these resources can be found in Table 4.

Designing a Therapy Regimen

A therapy regimen for asthma should be designed to help a patient gain control of his or her asthma. Based on the Expert Panel Report 2, there are two approaches to gaining control of asthma; both are based on the stepwise approach to asthma treatment outlined in the guidelines. The four steps of asthma and their definitions were introduced in unit 1 of this module. You will find these steps outlined in **Figure 3**. The two approaches to gaining control of disease are:
- Step down: Aim high, gain control, gain patient confidence, and then step down therapy as needed. In this approach, more aggressive therapy is initiated. Therapy is targeted a step above the patient's symptoms to gain rapid disease control. Once control is achieved, therapy can be backed down a step. Control is usually achieved with the use of oral corticosteroids or increased doses of inhaled corticosteroid. The Expert Panel Report 2 recommends this method.
- Step up: Start treatment at the step that corresponds with the severity of the patient's disease and then, if control is not achieved, gradually increase therapy to gain control.

In either case, once symptoms have been under control for several weeks or months, therapy should be reduced to minimal doses that control symptoms. The last medication added to the regimen should be the first medication to be gradually reduced to the lowest effective dose. In the case of inhaled corticosteroids, patients will most likely need to continue daily therapy, but the dose should be reduced to the lowest dose that controls symptoms. When a patient experiences an increase in symptoms, doses can be increased accordingly. The Expert Panel Report 2 recommendations for stepwise management and control of asthma in children >5 years old and adults based on symptom severity are provided in **Figure 4**. **Figure 5** provides an outline for treatment of pediatric patients <5 years old. In-depth discussion of the stepwise approach to therapy can be found in the Expert Panel Report 2 guidelines. These guidelines call for use of an anti-inflammatory agent in any patient with persistent asthma.

Stepwise approach for managing asthma in adults and children >5 years of age

Goals of Asthma Treatment

- ❏ Prevent chronic and troublesome symptoms (e.g., coughing or breathlessness in the night, in the early morning, or after exertion)
- ❏ Maintain (near) "normal" pulmonary function
- ❏ Maintain normal activity levels (including exercise and other physical activity)
- ❏ Prevent recurrent exacerbations of asthma and minimize the need for emergency department visits or hospitalizations
- ❏ Provide optimal pharmacotherapy with minimal or no adverse effects
- ❏ Meet patients' and families' expectations of and satisfaction with asthma care

CLASSIFY SEVERITY OF ASTHMA

Clinical Features Before Treatment[a]

	Symptoms[b]	Nighttime Symptoms	Lung Function
STEP 4 Severe Persistent	❏ Continual symptoms ❏ Limited physical activity ❏ Frequent exacerbations	Frequent	❏ FEV_1 or PEF <60% predicted ❏ PEF variability >30%
STEP 3 Moderate Persistent	❏ Daily symptoms ❏ Daily use of inhaled short-acting beta$_2$-adrenergic agonist ❏ Exacerbations affect activity ❏ Exacerbations >2 times a week; may last days	>1 time a week	❏ FEV_1 or PEF >60%–<80% predicted ❏ PEF variability >30%
STEP 2 Mild Persistent	❏ Symptoms >2 times a week but <1 time a day ❏ Exacerbations may affect activity	>2 times a month	❏ FEV_1 or PEF >80% predicted ❏ PEF variability 20–30%
STEP 1 Mild Intermittent	❏ Symptoms <2 times a week ❏ Asymptomatic and normal PEF between exacerbations ❏ Exacerbations brief (from a few hours to a few days); intensity may vary	<2 times a month	❏ FEV_1 or PEF >80% predicted ❏ PEF variability <20%

[a] The presence of one of the features of severity is sufficient to place a patient in that category. An individual should be assigned to the most severe grade in which any feature occurs. The characteristics noted in this figure are general and may overlap because asthma is highly variable. Furthermore, an individual's classification may change over time.

[b] Patients at any level of severity can have mild, moderate, or severe exacerbations. Some patients with intermittent asthma experience severe and life-threatening exacerbations separated by long periods of normal lung function and no symptoms.

Figure 3. Stepwise approach for managing asthma in adults and children >5 years of age
Source: reference 1.

Stepwise approach for treating asthma in adults and children >5 years of age based on symptom severity

	Long-Term Control	**Quick Relief**	**Education**
STEP 4 Severe Persistent	Daily medications: ❏ Anti-inflammatory: inhaled corticosteroid (high dose) AND ❏ Long-acting bronchodilator: either long-acting inhaled $beta_2$-adrenergic agonist, sustained-release theophylline, or long-acting $beta_2$-adrenergic agonist tablets AND ❏ Corticosteroid tablets or syrup long term (make repeat attempts to reduce systemic steroids and maintain control with high dose inhaled steroids)	❏ Short-acting bronchodilator: inhaled $beta_2$-adrenergic agonists as needed for symptoms. ❏ Intensity of treatment will depend on severity of exacerbation. ❏ Use of short-acting inhaled $beta_2$-adrenergic agonists on a daily basis, or increasing use, indicates the need for additional long-term-control therapy.	Steps 2 and 3 actions plus: ❏ Refer to individual education/counseling
STEP 3 Moderate Persistent	Daily medication: ❏ Either Anti-inflammatory: inhaled corticosteroid (medium dose) OR Inhaled corticosteroid (low-medium dose) and add a long-acting bronchodilator, especially for nighttime symptoms; either long-acting inhaled $beta_2$-adrenergic agonist, sustained-release theophylline, or long-acting $beta_2$-adrenergic agonist tablets. ❏ If needed Anti-inflammatory: inhaled corticosteroids (medium-high dose) AND Long-acting bronchodilator, especially for nighttime symptoms; either long-acting inhaled $beta_2$-adrenergic agonist, sustained-release theophylline, or long-acting $beta_2$-adrenergic agonist tablets.	❏ Short-acting bronchodilator: inhaled $beta_2$-adrenergic agonists as needed for symptoms. ❏ Intensity of treatment will depend on severity of exacerbation. ❏ Use of short-acting inhaled $beta_2$-adrenergic agonists on a daily basis, or increasing use, indicates the need for additional long-term-control therapy.	Step 1 actions plus: ❏ Teach self-monitoring ❏ Refer to group education if available ❏ Review and update self-management plan

	Long-Term Control	**Quick Relief**	**Education**
STEP 2 Mild Persistent	One daily medication: ☐ Anti-inflammatory: either inhaled corticosteroid (low doses) or cromolyn or nedocromil (children usually begin with a trial of cromolyn or nedocromil). ☐ Sustained-release theophylline to serum concentration of 5–15 mcg/mL is an alternative, but not preferred, therapy. Zafirlukast or zileuton may also be considered for patients >12 years of age, although their position in therapy is not fully established.	☐ Short-acting bronchodilator: inhaled beta$_2$-adrenergic agonists as needed for symptoms. ☐ Intensity of treatment will depend on severity of exacerbation. ☐ Use of short-acting inhaled beta$_2$-adrenergic agonists on a daily basis, or increasing use, indicates the need for additional long-term-control therapy.	Step 1 actions plus: ☐ Teach self-monitoring ☐ Refer to group education if available ☐ Review and update self-management plan
STEP 1 Mild Intermittent	☐ No daily medication needed.	☐ Short-acting bronchodilator: inhaled beta$_2$-adrenergic agonists as needed for symptoms. ☐ Intensity of treatment will depend on severity of exacerbation. ☐ Use of short-acting inhaled beta$_2$-adrenergic agonists more than 2 times a week may indicate the need to initiate long-term-control therapy.	☐ Teach basic facts about asthma ☐ Teach inhaler/spacer/holding chamber technique ☐ Discuss roles of medications ☐ Develop self-management plan ☐ Develop action plan for when and how to take rescue actions, especially for patients with a history of severe exacerbations ☐ Discuss appropriate environmental control measures to avoid exposure to known allergens and irritants

General Principles

Step down
Review treatment every 1 to 6 months; a gradual stepwise reduction in treatment may be possible.

Step up
If control is not maintained, consider step up. First, review patient medication technique, adherence, and environmental control (avoidance of allergens or other factors that contribute to asthma severity).

NOTE:
☐ The stepwise approach presents general guidelines to assist clinical decisionmaking; it is not intended to be a specific prescription. Asthma is highly variable; clinicians should tailor specific medication plans to the needs and circumstances of individual patients.
☐ Gain control as quickly as possible; then decrease treatment to the least medication necessary to maintain control. Gaining control may be accomplished by either starting treatment at the step most appropriate to the initial severity of the condition or starting at a higher level of therapy (e.g., a course of systemic corticosteroids or higher dose of inhaled corticosteroids).
☐ A rescue course of systemic corticosteroids may be needed at any time and at any step.
☐ Some patients with intermittent asthma experience severe and life-threatening exacerbations separated by long periods of normal lung function and no symptoms. This may be especially common with exacerbations provoked by respiratory infections. A short course of systemic corticosteroids is recommended.
☐ At each step, patients should control their environment to avoid or control factors that make their asthma worse (e.g., allergens, irritants); this requires specific diagnosis and education.
☐ Referral to an asthma specialist for consultation or comanagement is recommended if there are difficulties achieving or maintaining control of asthma or if the patient requires step 4 care. Referral may be considered if the patient requires step 3 care.

Figure 4. Stepwise approach for treating asthma in adults and children >5 years of age based on symptom severity
Source: reference 1.

Stepwise approach for treating infants and young children (5 years of age and younger) with acute or chronic asthma symptoms

	Long-Term Control	**Quick Relief**
STEP 4 Severe Persistent	❏ Daily anti-inflammatory medicine — High-dose inhaled corticosteroid with spacer/holding chamber and face mask — If needed, add systemic corticosteroids 2 mg/kg/day and reduce to lowest daily or alternate-day dose that stabilizes symptoms	❏ Bronchodilator as needed for symptoms (see step 1) up to 3 times a day
STEP 3 Moderate Persistent	❏ Daily anti-inflammatory medication. Either: — Medium-dose inhaled corticosteroid with spacer/holding chamber and face mask OR, once control is established: — Medium-dose inhaled corticosteroid and nedocromil OR — Medium-dose inhaled corticosteroid and long-acting bronchodilator (theophylline)	❏ Bronchodilator as needed for symptoms (see step 1) up to 3 times a day
STEP 2 Mild Persistent	❏ Daily anti-inflammatory medication. Either: — Cromolyn (nebulizer is preferred; or MDI) or nedocromil (MDI only) — Infants and young children usually begin with a trial of cromolyn or nedocromil OR — Low-dose inhaled corticosteroid with spacer/holding chamber and face mask	❏ Bronchodilator as needed for symptoms (see step 1)
STEP 1 Mild Intermittent	❏ No daily medication needed.	❏ Bronchodilator as needed for symptoms <2 times a week. Intensity of treatment will depend upon severity of exacer-bation. Either: — Inhaled short-acting beta$_2$-adrenergic agonist by nebulizer or face mask and spacer/holding chamber OR — Oral beta$_2$-adrenergic agonist for symptoms ❏ With viral respiratory infection — Bronchodilator every 4–6 hours up to 24 hours (longer with physician consult) but, in general, repeat no more than once every 6 weeks — Consider systemic corticosteroid if • Current exacerbation is severe OR • Patient has history of previous severe exacerbations

General Principles

Step down
↓ Review treatment every 1–6 months. If control is sustained for at least 3 months, a gradual stepwise reduction in treatment may be possible.

Step up
↑ If control is not achieved, consider step up. But first: review patient medication technique, adherence, and environmental control (avoidance of allergens or other precipitant factors).

NOTE:
- ❏ The stepwise approach presents guidelines to assist clinical decisionmaking. Asthma is highly variable; clinicians should tailor specific medication plans to the needs and circumstances of individual patients.
- ❏ Gain control as quickly as possible; then decrease treatment to the least medication necessary to maintain control. Gaining control may be accomplished by either starting treatment at the step most appropriate to the initial severity of their condition or by starting at a higher level of therapy (e.g., a course of systemic corticosteroids or higher dose of inhaled corticosteroids).
- ❏ A rescue course of systemic corticosteroid (prednisolone) may be needed at any time and step.
- ❏ In general, use of short-acting beta$_2$-adrenergic agonist on a daily basis indicates the need for additional long-term-control therapy.
- ❏ It is important to remember that there are very few studies on asthma therapy for infants.
- ❏ Consultation with an asthma specialist is recommended for patients with moderate or severe persistent asthma in this age group. Consultation should be considered for all patients with mild persistent asthma.

Figure 5. Stepwise approach for treating infants and young children (5 years of age and younger) with acute or chronic asthma symptoms
Source: reference 1.

The doses and numbers of medications may vary based on the patient's symptoms and level of control. Therapy may be stepped up as needed to regain control. Patients with intermittent disease, including exercise-induced bronchospasm (EIB), will most likely require a short-acting beta$_2$-adrenergic agonist to relieve or prevent symptoms. Pharmacologic management can be increased if symptoms become more persistent in nature and the short-acting beta$_2$-adrenergic agonist is needed more often than twice weekly for control of symptoms not associated with EIB or a concurrent viral illness. The recommendations of the Expert Panel Report 2 are general guidelines for therapy, and each clinician will need to tailor them to meet the specific needs of each individual patient. As you design a therapy regimen for a patient you will need to keep several factors in mind. These factors are listed in unit 13 of the *Core Module*, Figure 1.

Case Study

Let's go back to the case of Jeremy and design a therapy regimen for his asthma. Based on his symptoms and peak flow measurements he currently has moderate-persistent asthma. His old regimen can be found in unit 4, Appendix B and unit 5, Appendix C. Remember that Jeremy has had difficulty adhering to a medication regimen. He already has a prescription for albuterol and a prescription for Azmacort. From your interview you note that he has difficulty with nighttime symptoms. The APCP completed through the recommendation for therapy column can be found in **Appendix A**. To improve Jeremy's asthma control, the pharmacist makes these recommendations:

- change Azmacort 8 puffs four times daily to Pulmicort 1 puff twice daily; use with a spacer
- add Salmeterol (Serevent) 2 puffs at bedtime
- continue albuterol 2 puffs four times daily as needed
- discontinue albuterol nebulizer
- begin peak flow monitoring
- provide written daily self-management and action plan; developed jointly with patient
- provide instructions on inhaler, spacer, and peak flow meter technique
- re-evaluate patient in 2 weeks then again after another 2 weeks; then each month until stable

The pharmacist chose to change the inhaled corticosteroid to a product with increased potency that would require fewer puffs per day. Because Jeremy has significant nighttime symptoms, the pharmacist decided to initiate a long-acting beta$_2$-adrenergic agonist at bedtime. The albuterol will remain in Jeremy's regimen for acute symptom control. The use of a spacer was added to increase the deposition of medication in the lungs and decrease the potential of oral deposition and thrush. The pharmacist needs to contact the primary health care provider to suggest these changes to Jeremy's regimen. Jeremy has not been to see his primary care provider for asthma care in the past several months and as he has had numerous emergency rooms visits resulting from this disjointed care. Dr. Lefton appreciated the pharmacist's evaluation and decided to implement the changes.

Practice Example

Turn to the case of Sarah Jacobs, in **Appendix B**. Review the completed database forms. Sarah is 4 years old and newly diagnosed with mild-persistent asthma. She has had several wheezing episodes over the past 2 years associated with viral illness. The wheezing and coughing became more persistent this past spring. Her physician works with you in the clinic and has asked you to recommend a therapy regimen for Sarah. Complete the fourth column of the APCP found in Appendix B. You also need to develop an educational plan for Sarah and her family. What role will asthma education play in Sarah's treatment? What types of educational resources are available to Sarah? A completed APCP and sample educational plan for Sarah can be found in **Appendix C**.

The regimen chosen is:
- nedocromil (Tilade), started at four times per day and reduced to two times per day with symptom improvement, and
- albuterol 2 puffs four times daily as needed, used with face mask and holding chamber.

Summary

In this unit you have learned a great deal of information, including factors that affect the design of a therapy regimen and educational plan for a patient with asthma. Many educational resources are available to help you develop an educational program for your patients. Education is not a one-time activity, but one that must be reinforced with every patient encounter. The therapy regimen for a patient with asthma will be dynamic, changing as the patient's symptoms increase or decrease. Patients must understand their daily self-management plan and action plan. The pharmacist needs to serve as an educator and coach to help patients control their asthma.

References

1. National Heart, Lung, and Blood Institute. Expert Panel Report 2: Guidelines for the Diagnosis and Management of Asthma. July, 1997.
2. American Pharmaceutical Association. APhA Special Report. Asthma: The Pharmacist's Role in Optimizing Drug Delivery and Patient Compliance. Washington, DC: American Pharmaceutical Association; 1997. p. 21.
3. Powell CV, Everard ML. Treatment of childhood asthma: options and rationale for inhaled therapy. *Drugs* 1998; 55:237–52.

Self-Study Questions

Objective
Explain how patient-related concerns unique to patients with asthma may influence the design of their therapy regimens.

1. Explain how patient-related concerns unique to patients with asthma may influence decisions about the design of their therapy regimen.

2. Explain why a patient's perception of his or her disease needs to be considered when making decisions about the design of their therapy regimen.

3. Explain what considerations need to be incorporated into the design of a pediatric asthma patient's therapy regimen.

Objective
Explain the use of treatment guidelines in the design of therapy regimens for patients with asthma.

4. Explain the use of treatment guidelines in the design of therapy regimens for patients with asthma.

5. Appropriate use of treatment guidelines requires that you do which of the following?
   A. Follow each guideline exactly.
   B. Inform your asthma patients of the guidelines.
   C. Educate fellow health care workers about the guidelines.
   D. Remain aware of the currency of the guidelines.

6. In addition to national guidelines, pharmacists should be aware of specific guidelines used by all of the following *except*:
   A. the institution in which you work
   B. insurers
   C. individual patient families
   D. physician groups

Objective
Explain education needs unique to ambulatory care patients with asthma.

7. Name and describe education needs unique to ambulatory care patients with asthma.

8. All of the following should be an educational component for ambulatory asthma patients *except*:
   A. environmental control measures
   B. inhaler techniques
   C. medications and their role
   D. nutrition counseling

Objective
Explain factors unique to patients with asthma that affect the approaches used for education.

9. Name and explain each factor unique to patients with asthma that affect the choice of approaches for education related to the pharmacist's care plan.

10. The Internet can be a useful approach to patient education for the asthma patient.
    A. true
    B. false

Objective
Explain what is unique about the role of preventive education in patient-specific education for patients with asthma.

11. Explain what is unique about the role of preventive education in patient-specific education for patients with asthma.

Objective
State potential education resources used to meet an asthma patient's educational needs so the patient may successfully participate in the pharmacist's care plan.

12. List patient-specific education resources that meet an asthma patient's needs for learning to successfully participate in the pharmacist's care plan.

Objective
Design a therapy regimen, including patient-specific education, that meets the pharmacotherapeutic and related health care goals established for a patient with asthma, integrates patient disease-specific and drug information as well as ethical and quality-of-life issues, and considers pharmacoeconomic principles.

Self-Study Questions (cont.)

13. Refer to the case of Marie Cowling (unit 4, Appendixes F; unit 5, Appendix E; and unit 7, Appendix E). Then design a therapy regimen, including patient-specific education, for this patient. Record your answers in **Appendix D**.

Self-Study Answers

1. Depending on the specific patient-related concerns, adjustments in therapeutic plans need to be instituted. Patients' perceptions and beliefs about asthma will determine if they will be adherent and how aggressively they will manage their disease. Pediatric and elderly patients will have a confounding factor—a caregiver—that should be considered in the design. Environmental triggers need to be identified and patients must learn to avoid these triggers when possible. Ability to self-administer medication is also a unique concern for patients with arthritis or other physical disabilities and school-age children.

2. Patients who do not perceive asthma as life-threatening will be less likely to actively manage their disease and adhere to therapy recommendations.

3. Pediatric patients will most likely not be in control of their medications, but will depend on a caregiver or parent. The caregiver needs to be reliable and understand the need for medication adherence, environment control, and identification of worsening symptoms. Scheduling medication doses to occur outside of school will help the patient feel less conspicuous. Accessory devices (e.g., spacers and holding chambers) may be necessary for medication administration.

4. The Expert Panel Report 2 outlines the level of evidence for the management of asthma. When using guidelines, you must consider how current they are; you must also consider institution-specific guidelines and patient-specific needs.

5. D
6. C
7. Education needs include:
   - asthma overview: basic facts, stress and psychosocial adjustment, family involvement and social support, and exercise and activity;
   - medications and their role;
   - skills: inhaler technique (spacer/holding chamber use) and self-monitoring (use of peak flow meter);
   - environmental control measures;
   - rescue medication action plan: should include written daily self-management plan and action plan; and
   - use of health care systems and community resources.

8. D
9. Level of patient education; cognitive ability; literacy; language comprehension; vision; hearing; physical limitations; age
10. A
11. Asthma is a variable disease and is usually episodic in nature. Prevention of airway inflammation is at the center of asthma management. Patients need to be taught to manage their disease and prevent airway inflammation. Education about asthma, symptoms, triggers, environmental control, and prophylactic medication regimen adherence all stem from prevention of symptoms.

12. Education resources include:
    - American Lung Association (1-800-LUNG-USA; www.lungusa.org); validated educational programs ("Open Airways at School"); other educational pieces; multi-language
    - Asthma and Allergy Foundation of America (1-800-7-ASTHMA/www.aafa.org); validated educational programs ("Asthma Training Care for Kids" and "You Can Control Asthma"); other educational pieces; multi-language
    - National Technical Information Service (1-703-487-4650); validated educational programs ("Air Power," "Air Wise," "Living with Asthma," and "Open Airways"); other educational pieces; multi-language
    - National Asthma Education and Prevention Program (1-301-251-1222/ www.nhlbi.nih.gov/nhlbi/nhlbi.htm); validated educational program; other educational materials; multi-language
    - Allergy and Asthma Network/Mothers of Asthmatics, Inc. (1-800-878-4403/ www.aanma.com); educational resources
    - American Academy of Allergy, Asthma, and Immunology (1-800-822-ASTHMA/ www.aaaai.org); educational resources
    - American College of Allergy, Asthma, and Immunology (1-800-842-7777/ www.allergy.mcg.edu); educational programs

Self-Study Answers (cont.)

- National Jewish Medical and Research Center (1-800-222-LUNG/www.njc.org); educational programs
- American Association for Respiratory Care (1-972-243-2272)
- Healthy Kids: The Key to the Basics (1-617-965-9637)
- Pharmaceutical manufacturers

13. Refer to the APCP for Marie Cowling in **Appendix E**.

Ambulatory Pharmacist's Care Plan

Patient: Jeremy Morgan Pharmacist: Jennifer Loudon Date: March 10, 1999

DATE IDENTIFIED	PROBLEM (TPL)	PHARMACOTHERAPEUTIC AND RELATED HEALTH CARE GOAL	RECOMMENDATIONS FOR THERAPY	MONITORING PARAMETER(S)	DESIRED ENDPOINT(S)	MONITORING FREQUENCY
3/99	overuse of Albuterol	minimize symptoms optimize therapeutic regimen	D/C Neb solution Institute Serevent 2 puffs @ HS			
	intermittent refill record Azmacort	optimize education & medication administration	Δ to Pulmicort 1 puff BID			
	cigarette & alcohol use	protect confidentiality while educating about risks	Education			
	self-monitoring not done	Add peak flow monitoring	Daily PEF & Diary			
	poor symptom recognition	Educate about symptoms	Education			
	Echinacea use for prolonged time	Discontinue Echinacea	Discontinue			
	Influenza vaccine: Not vaccinated	Vaccinate yearly	Vaccinate in the fall			
	Misconceptions about corticosteroids	Provide Education	Education			

© 2000, American Society of Health-System Pharmacists, Inc. All rights reserved.

Pharmacist's Patient Database Form

Original Date: **4/6/99**
Date updated: _____
Date updated: _____
Date updated: _____

Demographic and Administrative Information

- **Name:** Sarah Jacobs
- **Social Security #:** 444-11-4444
- **Address:** 333 Mighty Oak Lane
- **Health Care Provider's Name:** Dr. Barker
- **Health Care Provider's Phone:** 663-6383
- **Work Phone:** N/A
- **Home Phone:** 262-5506 (Mom)
- **Date of Birth:** 3/12/95
- **Race:** White
- **Gender:** F
- **Religion:** N/A
- **Occupation:** Preschool
- **Health Insurer:** Magnicaring Plan
- **Subscriber #:** 444-11-4444-03
- **Primary Card Holder:** Frank
- **Drug Benefit:** ☐ yes ☒ no   copay: $_____

Current Symptoms

Wheezing/coughing

Past Medical History

wheezing c̄ viral illness × 2 years

Acute and Current Medical Problems

1. Asthma (new diagnosis)
2.
3.
4.
5.
6.
7.
8.

Family/Social/Economic History

Parents divorced – Dad remarried × 1 yr. (Frank)
Mom – Jane
Shared custody

Cost of medications per month $ N/A

Personal Limitations

None

Allergies/Intolerances NKDA

☒ No known drug allergies

Medication	Reaction

Social Drug Use   N/A

- Alcohol
- Caffeine
- Tobacco

Pregnancy/Breastfeeding Status

☐ Pregnant (due _____)   ☐ Breastfeeding

Diet

- ☐ Low salt
- ☐ Low fat
- ☐ Diabetic

Timing of meals:

Routine Exercise/Recreation

Daily Activities/Timing

Patient Name: **Sarah Jacobs**

Physical Assessment/Laboratory Data—Initial/Follow-up

Date	4/6/99				
Height					
Weight	30 lbs.				
Temp					
BP					
Pulse					
Respirations	20				
Peak Flow					
FBG					
R. Glucose					
HbA_{1c}					
T. Chol.					
LDL					
HDL					
TG					
INR					
BUN					
Cr					
ALT					
AST					
Alk Phos					

Drug Serum Concentrations

Date					

Notes:

© 2000, American Society of Health-System Pharmacists, Inc. All rights reserved.

Patient Name: Sarah Jacobs

Current Prescription Medication Regimen

Name/Dose/Strength/Route	Schedule/Frequency of Use	Indication	Start Date (and Stop Date If Applicable)	Prescriber	Adherence Issues/Efficacy

Current Nonprescription Medication Regimen (OTC, herbal, homeopathic, nutritional, etc.)

Name/Dose/Strength/Route	Schedule/Frequency of Use	Indication	Start Date (and Stop Date If Applicable)	Prescriber	Adherence Issues/Efficacy
Flintstones Chewable Vitamin	1 qd	supplement	~1 year	∅	∅
Tylenol Chewable Tabs	3 prn	fever	N/A		

Patient Name: **Sarah Jacobs**

Risk Assessment/Preventive Measures/Quality of Life

Cardiovascular Risk Assessment			
male >45 years old		1	
female >55 years old or female <55 with history of ovarectomy not taking estrogen replacement		1	
Definite MI or sudden death before age 55 year in father or male first-degree relative or before 65 year in mother or female first-degree relative	**N/A**	1	
current cigarette smoking		1	
hypertension		1	
diabetes mellitus		1	
HDL cholesterol <35 mg/dl		1	
HDL cholesterol >60 mg/dl		-1	
		Total:	

Is patient at risk for complications of current conditions? ☒ Yes ☐ No
Specify: **Morbidity and mortality from exacerbation of disease**

Preventive Measures for Adults H = has been done R = patient refuses X = not applicable		Date **4/6/99**		
Women				
Pap Smear/pelvic	Annually 19+			
Mammogram	Every 1-2Y 40-49; annually 50+			
Men				
Rectal/prostate	Annually 50+			
All Patients				
Total/HDL-C	Every 5Y 19+			
Home Fecal Occult Blood Test	Annually		**UTD**	
Immunizations				
Td	Every 10Y **(doesn't get, will need)**			
Influenza	Every fall*			
Pneumovax	Once*			

* if indicated

Quality of life issues
Parents divorced - shuffled back and forth between households

© 2000, American Society of Health-System Pharmacists, Inc. All rights reserved.

Assessment of General Appearance

Patient **Sarah Jacobs** _____ Date _____

General Appearance	Observations and Comments

Level of consciousness
   alertness: alert, confused,
   delirious, stuporous, comatose,
   orientation: person, place, time
	Alert + oriented x3

Signs of distress respiratory distress, pain, anxiety, etc.	None at present
Posture, motor activity, and gait *Describe*	Normal gait + posture
Dress, grooming, and personal hygiene *Describe*	Appropriate

Affect
   normal, inappropriate
   Describe
	Normal, slightly nervous

Speech
   normal, impaired
   Describe
	Normal

Skin
   color: normal, blue, brown, red, pallor
   texture: normal, coarse, dry, oily
   turgor: good, poor
   edema
   lesions: color, type, configuration, anatomic
      distribution, consistency
	Normal

Ambulatory Therapy Assessment Worksheet (ATAW)

Patient **Sarah Jacobs**
Pharmacist **Bill Jelen R.Ph**
Date **9-15-98**

Correlation Between Drug Therapy and Medical Problems

ASSESSMENT	PRESENCE OF PROBLEM*	COMMENTS/NOTES
Any drugs without a medical indication? Any unidentified medications? Any untreated medical conditions? Do they require drug therapy?	(1.) A problem exists. 2. More information is needed for determination. 3. No problem exists or an intervention is not needed.	Cromolyn used for diluent was DC'D

Appropriate Therapy

ASSESSMENT	PRESENCE OF PROBLEM*	COMMENTS/NOTES
Comparative efficacy of chosen medication(s)? Relative safety of chosen medication(s)? Is medication on formulary? Is nondrug therapy appropriately used (e.g., diet and exercise)? Is therapy achieving desired goals or outcomes? Is therapy tailored to this patient (e.g., age, comorbid conditions, and living/working environment)?	1. A problem exists. 2. More information is needed for determination. (3.) No problem exists or an intervention is not needed.	

Drug Regimen

ASSESSMENT	PRESENCE OF PROBLEM*	COMMENTS/NOTES
Are dose and dosing regimen appropriate and/or within usual therapeutic range and/or modified for patient factors? Appropriateness of PRN medications (prescribed or taken that way) Is route/dosage form/mode of administration appropriate? Does regimen and length or course of therapy consider efficacy, safety, convenience, patient limitations, and cost?	1. A problem exists. 2. More information is needed for determination. (3.) No problem exists or an intervention is not needed.	

*Problem denotes any pharmacotherapeutic or related health care problem.

© 2000, American Society of Health-System Pharmacists, Inc. All rights reserved.

Therapeutic Duplication

ASSESSMENT	PRESENCE OF PROBLEM*	COMMENTS/NOTES
Any therapeutic duplication?	1. A problem exists. 2. More information is needed for determination. **(3.)** No problem exists or an intervention is not needed.	

Drug Allergy or Intolerance

ASSESSMENT	PRESENCE OF PROBLEM*	COMMENTS/NOTES
Allergy or intolerance to any medications (or chemically related medications) currently being taken? Is patient using a method to alert health care providers of the allergy/intolerance or serious health problem?	**(1.)** A problem exists. 2. More information is needed for determination. 3. No problem exists or an intervention is not needed.	pt. continues to use DC'D cromolyn

Adverse Drug Events

ASSESSMENT	PRESENCE OF PROBLEM*	COMMENTS/NOTES
Are symptoms or medical problems drug induced? What is the likelihood the problem is drug related?	**(1.)** A problem exists. 2. More information is needed for determination. 3. No problem exists or an intervention is not needed.	continues DC'D Med more education needed

Interactions: Drug-Drug, Drug-Disease, Drug-Nutrient, Drug–Laboratory Test

ASSESSMENT	PRESENCE OF PROBLEM*	COMMENTS/NOTES
Any drug-drug interactions? Clinical significance? Any relative or absolute contraindications given patient characteristics and current/past disease states? Any drug-nutrient interactions? Clinical significance? Any drug-laboratory test interactions? Clinical significance?	1. A problem exists. **(2.)** More information is needed for determination. 3. No problem exists or an intervention is not needed.	

*Problem denotes any pharmacotherapeutic or related health care problem.

© 2000, American Society of Health-System Pharmacists, Inc. All rights reserved.

Social or Recreational Drug Use

ASSESSMENT	PRESENCE OF PROBLEM*	COMMENTS/NOTES
Is current use of social drugs problematic? Are symptoms related to sudden withdrawal or discontinuation of social drugs?	(1.) A problem exists. 2. More information is needed for determination. 3. No problem exists or an intervention is not needed.	inhaled steriod and cromolyn

Financial Impact

ASSESSMENT	PRESENCE OF PROBLEM*	COMMENTS/NOTES
Is therapy cost-effective? Does cost of therapy represent a financial hardship for the patient?	1. A problem exists. 2. More information is needed for determination. (3.) No problem exists or an intervention is not needed.	

Patient Knowledge of Therapy

ASSESSMENT	PRESENCE OF PROBLEM*	COMMENTS/NOTES
Does patient understand the role of his/her medication(s), how to take it, and potential side effects? Would patient benefit from education tools (e.g., written patient education sheets, wallet cards, or reminder package?) Does the patient understand the role of nondrug therapy?	1. A problem exists. 2. More information is needed for determination. (3.) No problem exists or an intervention is not needed.	

Adherence

ASSESSMENT	PRESENCE OF PROBLEM*	COMMENTS/NOTES
Is there a problem with nonadherence to drug or nondrug therapy (e.g., diet and exercise)? Are there barriers to adherence or factors hindering the achievement of therapeutic efficacy?	1. A problem exists. 2. More information is needed for determination. (3.) No problem exists or an intervention is not needed.	

*Problem denotes any pharmacotherapeutic or related health care problem.

© 2000, American Society of Health-System Pharmacists, Inc. All rights reserved.

Self-Monitoring

ASSESSMENT	PRESENCE OF PROBLEM*	COMMENTS/NOTES
Does patient perform appropriate self-monitoring? (e.g., peak flow and blood glucose) Is correct technique employed? Is self-monitoring performed consistently, at appropriate times, and with appropriate frequency?	1. A problem exists. **(2.)** More information is needed for determination. 3. No problem exists or an intervention is not needed.	

Risks and Quality of Life Impacts

ASSESSMENT	PRESENCE OF PROBLEM*	COMMENTS/NOTES
Is patient at risk for complications with an existing disease state (i.e., risk factor assessment)? Is patient on track for preventive measures (e.g., immunizations, mammograms, prostate exams, eye exams)? Is therapy adversely impacting patient's quality of life? How so?	1. A problem exists. 2. More information is needed for determination. **(3.)** No problem exists or an intervention is not needed.	

*Problem denotes any pharmacotherapeutic or related health care problem.

© 2000, American Society of Health-System Pharmacists, Inc. All rights reserved.

Ambulatory Pharmacist's Care Plan

Patient: Sarah Jacobs Pharmacist: Bill Jelen Date: 4-99

DATE IDENTIFIED	PROBLEM (TPL)	PHARMACOTHERAPEUTIC AND RELATED HEALTH CARE GOAL	RECOMMENDATIONS FOR THERAPY	MONITORING PARAMETER(S)	DESIRED ENDPOINT(S)	MONITORING FREQUENCY
4/6/99	New diagnosis asthma-associated w/viral illness	control of sxs				
4/6	Basic asthma education needed	Education				
4/6	No flu vaccine	vaccination in fall				

© 2000, American Society of Health-System Pharmacists, Inc. All rights reserved.

Ambulatory Pharmacist's Care Plan

Patient ___Sarah Jacobs___ Pharmacist ___Bill Jelen___ Date ___4-99___

DATE IDENTIFIED	PROBLEM (TPL)	PHARMACOTHERAPEUTIC AND RELATED HEALTH CARE GOAL	RECOMMENDATIONS FOR THERAPY	MONITORING PARAMETER(S)	DESIRED ENDPOINT(S)	MONITORING FREQUENCY
4/6/99	New diagnosis asthma-associated w/viral illness	control of sxs	Tilade 2 puffs qid Albuterol qid prn			
4/6	Basic asthma education needed	Education	Set up education plan—will need to include both parents			
4/6	No flu vaccine	vaccination in fall	schedule in fall			

Educational Plan for Sarah Jacobs

Education of child and parents on basics of asthma, medication use and role, environmental control, daily symptom management; inhaler technique and spacer technique; symptom recognition; and skills.

Child caregiver also needs to understand the basics of asthma and role of education. Will need to reinforce with parents the need for daily treatment to prevent exacerbations.

Ambulatory Pharmacist's Care Plan

Patient: Marie Cowling   Pharmacist: Jim Bellows   Date: July 8, 1999

DATE IDENTIFIED	PROBLEM (TPL)	PHARMACOTHERAPEUTIC AND RELATED HEALTH CARE GOAL	RECOMMENDATIONS FOR THERAPY	MONITORING PARAMETER(S)	DESIRED ENDPOINT(S)	MONITORING FREQUENCY
7/8/99	Overuse of Beta-adrenergic agonist	Use Beta-adrenergic agonist appropriately & have good disease control				
	No local health care provider	Establish relationship with local physician				
	No PEF monitoring	PEF monitoring				
	Possible drug-disease interaction	No drug-disease interaction				
	Improved disease control	Asthma control				
↓	Arthritis	Control of arthritis symptoms				

Ambulatory Pharmacist's Care Plan

Patient __Marie Cowling__   Pharmacist __Jim Bellows__   Date __July 1999__

DATE IDENTIFIED	PROBLEM (TPL)	PHARMACOTHERAPEUTIC AND RELATED HEALTH CARE GOAL	RECOMMENDATIONS FOR THERAPY	MONITORING PARAMETER(S)	DESIRED ENDPOINT(S)	MONITORING FREQUENCY
	Overuse of Beta-adrenergic agonist	Use Beta-adrenergic agonist appropriately & have good disease control	Add Aerobid 2 puffs BID ↓ use of Maxair use PRN			
	No local health care provider	Establish relationship with local physician	Refer to Joan Owens-social worker for MD Referral			
	No PEF monitoring	PEF monitoring	Daily PEF to establish personal best then periodic assessment			
	Possible drug-disease interaction	No drug-disease interaction	DC ibuprofen use Tylenol for osteoarthritis pain			
	improved disease control	Asthma control	patient education identify trigger patient will need symptom diary			
	Arthritis	control of arthritis symptoms	DC ibuprofen use Tylenol for osteoarthritis pain			

© 2000, American Society of Health-System Pharmacists, Inc. All rights reserved.

Ambulatory Pharmacist's Care Plan

Patient __Mary Franklin__   Pharmacist __Cheryl Marks__   Date __9/20/99__

DATE IDENTIFIED	PROBLEM (TPL)	PHARMACOTHERAPEUTIC AND RELATED HEALTH CARE GOAL	RECOMMENDATIONS FOR THERAPY	MONITORING PARAMETER(S)	DESIRED ENDPOINT(S)	MONITORING FREQUENCY
9/20/99	Overuse of Beta-adrenergic agonist	Appropriate use & maintain disease control				
	No local provider	Local health care provider identified				
	No PEF monitoring	Daily PEF reading to establish personal best & periodic				
	Baseline Education	Understanding of medication use and disease				
	Asthma poorly controlled	Education medication management				

Designing a Monitoring Plan for Patients with Asthma

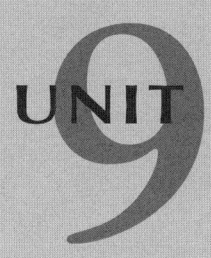

UNIT 9

Unit Objectives	236
Unit Organization	236
Unique Issues in Monitoring Therapy for Ambulatory Care Patients with Asthma	236
Determining Parameters to Measure Achievement of Pharmacotherapeutic and Related Health Care Goals	236
Drug Characteristics	236
Determining Desired Measurable Values for Monitoring Parameters	238
Example Case	239
Factors Influencing the Frequency and Timing of Parameter Measurements	239
Designing a Monitoring Plan for an Ambulatory Care Patient with Asthma— Case Study	239
Practice Example	240
Summary	240
Reference	240
Self-Study Questions	241
Self-Study Answers	243
Appendixes	244

In unit 8, you learned how to design a therapy regimen for an ambulatory care patient with asthma. The next step in the pharmacotherapeutic process is development of a monitoring plan that allows you to track your patient's progress and the outcomes of your therapy recommendations. To provide optimal therapy (i.e., pharmaceutical care), you need to know whether the desired outcomes have been achieved.

Unit Objectives

After you successfully complete this unit, you will be able to:
- state customary monitoring parameters for medication regimens commonly prescribed in the ambulatory care setting for patients with asthma,
- determine parameters to monitor that will measure achievement of pharmacotherapeutic and related health care goals for ambulatory care patients with asthma,
- determine desired measurable values for monitoring parameters in the treatment of patients with asthma in the ambulatory care setting,
- describe factors that should influence the frequency and timing of parameter measurements in monitoring plans for ambulatory care patients with asthma, and
- design a monitoring plan for a regimen for an ambulatory care patient with asthma that effectively evaluates achievement of pharmacotherapeutic and related health care goals.

Unit Organization

In this unit, you will learn to specify monitoring parameters, endpoints, and frequency of monitoring for the therapy of an ambulatory care patient with asthma. You then learn how this information is incorporated into a monitoring plan and the effect of treatment guidelines on the plan.

Unique Issues in Monitoring Therapy for Ambulatory Care Patients with Asthma

Determining Parameters to Measure Achievement of Pharmacotherapeutic and Related Health Care Goals

As you learned in unit 15 of the *Core Module*, you should consider several factors when selecting monitoring parameters, including:
- drug characteristics;
- therapeutic efficacy and adverse effects of regimen;
- physiological changes in the patient;
- practicality, availability, and cost of monitoring;
- patient adherence; and
- follow-up on referrals.

Unit 15 of the *Core Module* explains each of these factors in more detail; please review it as needed.

Drug Characteristics

With the exception of theophylline, medications used in the treatment of asthma do not require serum concentration monitoring. The therapeutic effectiveness of agents used to treat asthma is best assessed by evaluation of the patient's lung function (e.g., peak flow assessment and presence of airflow obstruction), symptoms, quality of life, school or job absenteeism, and patient satisfaction. Theophylline is indicated in patients with persistent asthma, but is not considered a first-choice therapy. Patients receiving theophylline do require occasional serum concentration monitoring. If theophylline is added to the regimen, serum concentrations ranging from 5 to 15 µg/ml are desired in most patients. Factors that would prompt you to evaluate a serum concentration (trough level suggested) include:
- adherence assessment,
- suspicion of toxicity,
- worsening disease,
- addition of medication that may interact,
- febrile illness (decreases theophylline clearance),
- smoking cessation, and
- dosing or formulation change.

Table 1. Potential Adverse Effects of Asthma Medications

Inhaled Corticosteroids	Cough, dysphonia, and oral thrush High doses: systemic effects
Systemic Corticosteroids	Long-term use: adrenal suppression, osteoporosis, growth suppression, skin thinning, bruising, hypertension, diabetes, Cushing's syndrome, and cataracts
	Short-term use: hyperglycemia, fluid retention, weight gain, increased appetite, mood changes, hypertension, GI distress, and ulcers
Cromolyn Sodium	Bronchospasm
Nedocromil	Unpleasant taste
Beta$_2$-adrenergic Agonists	Tachycardia, skeletal muscle tremor, hypokalemia, headache, hyperglycemia, and electrocardiogram changes on overdose (QT$_c$ prolongation)
Theophylline	GI upset, increased gastroesophageal reflux, CNS stimulation, insomnia, and urine retention in males with prostate inflammation
	Toxicity: tachycardia, nausea, vomiting, supraventricular tachycardia, headache, seizures, and hypokalemia
Montelukast	Headache and stomach upset
Zafirlukast	Headache and increased LFTs
Zileuton	Increased LFTs and GI upset
Ipratropium Bromide	Dry mouth and blurred vision

GI, gastrointestinal; CNS, central nervous system; LFTs, liver function tests.

Potential adverse effects of asthma medications can be found in **Table 1**. The presence or absence of adverse effects should be assessed in each patient. Use of medications that may cause liver toxicity, such as zileuton, requires periodic monitoring of liver function. Theophylline toxicity can be noted both by symptoms and by elevated serum concentrations. Remember that some patients may experience signs of toxicity within the therapeutic range.

The majority of your evaluation of therapeutic effectiveness in an asthma patient will be centered on these parameters:
- lung function,
- quality of life, and
- adverse drug effects/interactions.

Lung function can be assessed, as discussed in unit 3, by peak flow measurements, work of breathing assessment, direct auscultation, and patient-reported symptoms. Review the patient's peak flow measurements and have him or her demonstrate peak flow measurement during each encounter. Encourage patients to keep a daily diary to record their symptoms and need for rescue medications. Along with peak flow readings, this will be helpful for analyzing trends.

Quality-of-life assessment should include an evaluation of the number of encounters the patient has had with the health care system within a given period of time. Other questions that are useful in this assessment include:
- How often have asthma exacerbations disrupted the patient's life?
- What effect has asthma had on the patient's school, work, or social-function attendance?
- Are the medications or schedule of medications interfering with activities of daily living?
- Is travel restricted because of frequent exacerbations and the need to be close to a physician or other health care provider?
- Does the patient avoid visiting certain friends, buildings, or other establishments because the environment triggers symptoms?
- Does the patient not participate in sports, camps, or other physical activities because of symptoms?

Adverse drug effects or drug interactions should be assessed with each patient encounter. Always check to see if new medications have been added to the patient's regimen. Ask the patient if the medications are causing problems. Liver function tests (LFTs) are useful for evaluation of zileuton. Linear growth should be monitored in pediatric patients receiving corticosteroids. Although the potential for growth suppression is present, the benefit of treatment to the patient usually outweighs growth effects; however, pediatric corticosteroid therapy remains controversial because of the number of complications affecting growth in this population. In cases of suspected hypothalamic-pituitary-axis suppression from systemic corticosteroids or high doses of inhaled corticosteroids, ACTH stimulation tests may be warranted. A primary health care provider would most likely order these tests, although you may bring the concern to the attention of the health care practitioner.

The presence of adverse effects or disruptions to a patient's quality of life have a profound effect on adherence. Adherence can be difficult for patients but becomes especially burdensome when patients experience unpleasant effects from their medications. Refer to unit 15 of the *Core Module* for further discussion on adherence.

Determining Desired Measurable Values for Monitoring Parameters

Now that you have identified what parameters you would like to follow, you will need to identify what those values or responses should be. For example, what peak flow measurement would be acceptable for a patient with asthma? The Expert Panel Report 2 recommends that as patients' peak expiratory flow (PEF) measurement falls below 80% of their personal best, they should remain alert to worsening symptoms. PEF measurements have been separated into zones for the purpose of the patient's action plan:
- Green zone (good control) is usually defined as 80–100% of personal best PEF.
- Yellow zone (caution) is usually defined as 50–80% of personal best PEF.
- Red zone (medical alert) is usually defined as <50% of personal best PEF.

These numbers are arbitrary and may vary, depending on the clinician. Each step of the action plan will specify what action the patient should initiate based on symptoms and PEF values. Interventions in the yellow zone usually require that the patient step up therapy or add another medication. A patient in the red zone should increase medications, start oral corticosteroids, and contact his or her doctor or seek medical attention. Each patient will have an individualized action plan, based on his or her own goals and those of the primary health care provider.

Other goals in assessment of lung function are no evidence of wheezing or airway obstruction and minimal to no reports of symptoms. You want the patient to be free of nighttime symptoms and, ideally, have no need to use rescue therapy for acute exacerbations. Another goal is decreased absenteeism and the ability to participate in work, school, and social activities. Obviously, ideal goals will not be achievable for every asthma patient. Depending on the patient, your goal may be to simply reduce the number of exacerbations and missed school or work days. Some symptoms are to be expected in patients with more severe disease.

Ideally, you do not want a patient to experience adverse effects or symptoms. If a patient experiences an increase in LFT values as a result of leukotriene medications, the medication must be discontinued. However, if a patient experiences oral thrush from inhaled corticosteroids, the best approach would be to have the patient use a spacer or holding chamber for drug administration. Advising the patient to rinse his or her mouth with water after using the inhaled corticosteroid will also help decrease this adverse effect. Some adverse effects may be only slightly bothersome to the patient and may be acceptable when compared with the symptoms of disease. You need to discuss and individualize your approach to handling adverse effects with each patient. In some cases, the risk vs. benefit gained from the medication may dictate that the drug be discontinued. In other cases, the adverse effect may be minimal and therapy may be continued.

Example Case

Consider the case of Brian Marcs. Brian is a 25-year-old African American male with severe-persistent asthma. An ideal goal for Brian would be for him to be symptom free at all times. Based on his history, this would be an unrealistic goal. Currently, Brian experiences nighttime symptoms on a daily basis and requires urgent care treatment on a monthly basis. He also misses 2–3 days of college classes per quarter. Some goals for Brian might be to reduce his nighttime symptoms to no more than twice per week and to have no need for urgent care visits or missed school days. Brian will most likely need to step up his medications based on his PEF and symptoms. If Brian can gain more control of his disease, he may be able to improve his quality of life.

Factors Influencing the Frequency and Timing of Parameter Measurements

When evaluating a peak flow reading, be aware that the diurnal effect of cortisol release can affect the measured PEF. Patients should be instructed to measure their peak flow at consistent times of the day. Patients who are instructed to monitor their peak flow daily should do so in the morning when they wake up, before use of a beta$_2$-adrenergic agonist. A consistent morning hour will enable the patient to consistently monitor changes. Patients then recheck PEF as needed when symptoms worsen. Not all patients monitor peak flow measurements daily. The Expert Panel Report 2 recommends daily monitoring for patients with moderate-to-severe–persistent asthma. When patients are not motivated to complete daily monitoring, they may be instructed to record a personal best PEF. After 2–3 weeks of daily monitoring, the frequency is reduced to checking PEF periodically or as symptoms worsen.

Sometimes the frequency of monitoring is recommended by the manufacturer. For example, the frequency of LFT monitoring (for serum alanine aminotransferase [ALT]) in a patient receiving zileuton is recommended at the following times:
- before treatment begins,
- once a month for the first 3 months,
- every 2–3 months for the remainder of the first year, and
- periodically thereafter.

Patients who have signs of liver toxicity, flu-like symptoms, increases in their ALT concentrations, or jaundice need to be monitored more frequently if the drug is continued.

The frequency of monitoring is not always specified for each medication. Although it is recommended that theophylline levels are followed, the exact frequency of the monitoring will depend on the patient. You and your patient should use the criteria discussed in the first section of this unit as a guide to determine how frequently theophylline serum concentrations should be obtained.

As with any disease, patients may require more frequent monitoring of their asthma early in the course of therapy or while changing or titrating therapy. Patients with concomitant diseases and more complex therapy regimens will require more frequent monitoring.

A more detailed discussion regarding the determination of personal best peak flow readings can be found in unit 2 of this module.

Designing a Monitoring Plan for an Ambulatory Care Patient with Asthma— Case Study

Let's take another look at the case of Jeremy Morgan. Let's consider how we will monitor his progress toward meeting the stated pharmacotherapeutic and related health care goals. We will work through the completion of the APCP for Jeremy, as well as development of the Ambulatory Monitoring Worksheet (AMW) to track selected monitoring parameters. (His initial database can be found in unit 4, Appendix B; unit 5, Appendix A; unit 7, Appendix A; and unit 8, Appendix A.) A completed APCP and AMW can be found at the end of this unit, in **Appendix A**.

Jeremy came to the pharmacist's attention with a long history of asthma. His main goals concern the need to improve asthma control and prevent exacerbations. The first goal is to minimize symptoms and optimize his therapy regimen. Jeremy frequently suffers from nighttime symptoms, sleeps in an elevated position, and uses continuous albuterol nebulizers. The recommendation is to discontinue the albuterol nebulizer and begin salmeterol at bedtime. Monitoring parameters for this change in therapy will be to monitor the frequency and severity of nighttime symptoms and morning PEF readings. Jeremy should keep a symptom diary and monitor these parameters daily. The pharmacist should monitor the parameters with each visit.

Adherence has been an issue for Jeremy in the past. He and his mother both have expressed concerns about inhaled corticosteroids. Because Jeremy will continue to need inhaled corticosteroids, the pharmacist decided to optimize medications and provide education about inhaled corticosteroids. A therapy change from his present inhaled corticosteroid, triamcinolone, to budesonide was suggested. This change will reduce the number of inhalations per dose and the numbers of administration times per day. These changes should simplify Jeremy's regimen and increase adherence. Adherence and symptom control as well as peak flow readings and inhaler technique will be addressed during each visit. All other recommendations were addressed in the same manner, and monitoring parameters and frequency of monitoring were noted on the APCP. The majority of recommendations for Jeremy are interrelated, with overlapping monitoring parameters.

The monitoring parameters have been transferred to the AMW, with frequencies noted.

Practice Example

Refer to the case of 4-year-old Sarah Jacobs, introduced in unit 8, Appendixes B and C. Design a monitoring plan for Sarah using the APCP completed through recommendations for therapy and the blank AMW provided in **Appendix B**. When you have completed these, compare your responses to the author's, found in **Appendix C**.

Summary

Monitoring plans are designed to measure the achievement of pharmacotherapeutic and related health care goals established for a patient with asthma. You should begin by determining what parameters should be assessed, defining the target endpoint, and determining the frequency of monitoring for these parameters (outcomes). You will not be able to determine if a goal has been achieved if it has not been clearly defined ahead of time.

Reference

1. McEvoy GK. *AHFS 99 Drug Information*. Bethesda, MD: American Society of Health-System Pharmacists; 1999.

Self-Study Questions

Objective
State customary monitoring parameters for medication regimens commonly prescribed in the ambulatory care setting for patients with asthma.

1. List customary monitoring parameters for medication regimens commonly prescribed in the ambulatory care setting for patients with asthma.

Objective
Determine parameters to monitor that will measure achievement of pharmacotherapeutic and related health care goals for ambulatory care patients with asthma.

Refer to the case of Marie Cowling (**Appendix D**) for questions 2–4.

2. Which of the following best describes a monitoring parameter that will measure achievement of appropriate beta$_2$-adrenergic agonist use?
   A. report from physician
   B. weight of inhaler canister
   C. patient report of symptoms and refill history
   D. peak flow readings

3. Which of the following best describes a monitoring parameter that will measure achievement of peak flow monitoring?
   A. physician report
   B. refill history
   C. patient report and diary
   D. patient demonstration of technique

4. Which of the following best describes a monitoring parameter that will measure achievement of no drug-disease interaction (asthma and ibuprofen)?
   A. patient medication diary
   B. patient report of symptoms, to establish if ibuprofen causes exacerbation
   C. serum ibuprofen concentrations
   D. urinalysis

Refer to the case of Mike Kelley (unit 7, Appendix C) for questions 5–7.

5. Which of the following best describes a monitoring parameter that will measure the achievement of knowledge of disease management for Mr. Kelley.
   A. refill history
   B. physician report
   C. patient report
   D. peak flow monitor diary

6. Which of the following best describes a monitoring parameter that will measure improved disease management?
   A. patient report, ability to participate in activities, and decreased symptoms
   B. serum IgE concentrations
   C. peak flow monitoring
   D. employer report of improved productivity

7. Which of the following best describes a monitoring parameter that will measure Mr. Kelly's medication regimen adherence?
   A. patient report
   B. refill history
   C. technique demonstration
   D. peak flow diary

Objective
Determine desired measurable values for monitoring parameters in the treatment of patients with asthma in the ambulatory care setting.

Refer to the case of Marie Cowling for question 8.

8. Determine desired measurable values for monitoring parameters in the treatment of Marie Cowling.

Objective
Describe factors that should influence the frequency and timing of parameter measurements in monitoring plans for ambulatory care patients with asthma.

9. Explain how the presence of symptoms of an exacerbation would influence the frequency and timing of peak flow monitoring for ambulatory care patients with asthma.

10. Explain how the presence of nausea and vomiting would influence the frequency and

Self-Study Questions (cont.)

timing of theophylline serum concentration monitoring for ambulatory care patients with asthma.

11. Explain how diurnal effects of cortisol release influence the frequency and timing of peak flow measurements.

Objective
Design a monitoring plan for a regimen for an ambulatory care patient with asthma that effectively evaluates achievement of pharmacotherapeutic and related health care goals.

12. Using her APCP completed through the Recommendations for Therapy Column and the blank AMW in Appendix D, design a monitoring plan for Marie Cowling.

Self-Study Answers

1. refill history, frequency of symptoms, adverse effects from medications, peak flow measurements, urgent care and ER visits, nighttime symptoms, lung function, and quality of life

2. C

3. C

4. B

5. C

6. A

7. B

8. peak flow (she will need to determine personal best and then zone values will be determined for her) and refill history

9. Patients experiencing an acute exacerbation will monitor PEF more frequently to evaluate the effects of medications and look for decreased PEF and worsening exacerbations.

10. These symptoms could be a sign of toxicity; this would cause you to evaluate a serum concentration immediately.

11. Cortisol levels are lowest in the early morning (4:00 a.m.). Consistent measurement of PEF is suggested to evaluate trends in fluctuations. Suggestions are to check PEF in the morning on rising, before medication administration. This allows you to evaluate PEF when it is probably at its lowest point.

12. See Appendix E

Ambulatory Pharmacist's Care Plan

Patient: Jeremy Morgan   Pharmacist: Jennifer Loudon   Date: March 10, 1999

DATE IDENTIFIED	PROBLEM (TPL)	PHARMACOTHERAPEUTIC AND RELATED HEALTH CARE GOAL	RECOMMENDATIONS FOR THERAPY	MONITORING PARAMETER(S)	DESIRED ENDPOINT(S)	MONITORING FREQUENCY
3/99	overuse of Albuterol	minimize symptoms optimize therapeutic regimen	D/C Neb solution Institute Serevent 2 puffs @ HS	Frequency & severity of nighttime sx; monitor PEFS	PEFS >80% No morning dip in PEF. No nighttime symptoms	Each visit
	intermittent refill record Azmacort	optimize education & medication administration	Δ to 1 puff BID Pulmicort	PEF Refill hx symptom diary	Normal PEF No exacerbations adherence	Each visit
	cigarette & Alcohol use	protect confidentiality while educating about risks	Education	Patient report	No exposure	Each visit
	self-monitoring not done	Add peak flow monitoring	Daily PEF & Diary	Diary evaluation	Daily monitor	Each visit
	poor symptom recognition	Educate about symptoms	Education	Patient report	Recognition of symptoms	Each visit
	Echinacea use for prolonged time	Discontinue Echinacea	Discontinue	Patient/parent report	D/C	Each visit
	Influenza vaccine: Not vaccinated	Vaccinate yearly	Vaccinate in the fall	Patient records	vaccination	Every fall
	Misconceptions about corticosteroids	Provide Education	Education	Patient report adherence	adherence	Each visit

PHARMACIST'S CARE PLAN AMBULATORY MONITORING WORKSHEET (AMW)

Patient: Jeremy Morgan

Pharmacist: Jennifer Loudon
Date: 3/10/99

Pharmaco-therapeutic Goal	Monitoring Parameter	Desired Endpoint	Monitoring Frequency	Date 3/10/99													
Improve asthma control	Symptom Diary	↓ freq. of sx	q month														
	(refill hx) Beta-adrenergic agonist use	<1 canister per month	q month														
	(refill hx) Pulmicort use	No gaps in refill	q month														
↓	Nighttime Sx	None	(patient) Daily														
Monitoring of peak flow	Morning PEF	Daily ✓'s	(patient) Daily														
	Influenza vaccine	Given	q fall														
Education	Patient knowledge	Understanding	q visit														
↓	Inhaler technique	Appropriate	q visit														
Monitoring	Evening PEF	Daily ✓'s	q visit														
Cigarette & Alcohol Education	Patient/parent report	0 exposures	q visit														
d/c echinacea	Patient/parent report	D/C	q visit														

© 2000, American Society of Health-System Pharmacists, Inc. All rights reserved.

Ambulatory Pharmacist's Care Plan

Patient: Sarah Jacobs   Pharmacist: Bill Jelen   Date: 4-99

DATE IDENTIFIED	PROBLEM (TPL)	PHARMACOTHERAPEUTIC AND RELATED HEALTH CARE GOAL	RECOMMENDATIONS FOR THERAPY	MONITORING PARAMETER(S)	DESIRED ENDPOINT(S)	MONITORING FREQUENCY
4/6/99	New diagnosis asthma—associated w/viral illness	control of sxs	Tilade 2 puffs qid Albuterol qid prn			
4/6	Basic asthma education needed	Education	Set up education plan—will need to include both parents			
4/6 reaffirm 2/22	No flu vaccine	vaccination in fall	schedule in fall			

© 2000, American Society of Health-System Pharmacists, Inc. All rights reserved.

PHARMACIST'S CARE PLAN AMBULATORY MONITORING WORKSHEET (AMW)

Patient _____   Pharmacist _____
                                  Date _____

Pharmaco-therapeutic Goal	Monitoring Parameter	Desired Endpoint	Monitoring Frequency	Date												

© 2000, American Society of Health-System Pharmacists, Inc. All rights reserved.

Ambulatory Pharmacist's Care Plan

Patient __Sarah Jacobs__   Pharmacist __Bill Jelen__   Date __4-99__

DATE IDENTIFIED	PROBLEM (TPL)	PHARMACOTHERAPEUTIC AND RELATED HEALTH CARE GOAL	RECOMMENDATIONS FOR THERAPY	MONITORING PARAMETER(S)	DESIRED ENDPOINT(S)	MONITORING FREQUENCY
4/6/99	New diagnosis — asthma associated w/ viral illness	control of sxs	Tilade 2 puffs qid Albuterol qid prn	symptoms exacerbations refill hx gaps in refill	minimal sxs no exacerbations, appropriate refills	q visit q refill
4/6	Basic asthma education needed	Education	Set up education plan—will need to include both parents	✓ patient/parent understanding	patient/parent understanding pathophys & meds	q visit
4/6	No flu vaccine	vaccination in fall	schedule in fall	✓ if received	vaccinated	q fall

PHARMACIST'S CARE PLAN AMBULATORY MONITORING WORKSHEET (AMW)

Patient Sarah Jacobs

Pharmacist Bill Jelen

Date 4-6-99

Pharmaco-therapeutic Goal	Monitoring Parameter	Desired Endpoint	Monitoring Frequency	Date												
Asthma control	Symptom diary	No symptoms	q visit													
Med adherence	Albuterol refill hx	<1 canister per month	q visit													
Med adherence	Tilade refill hx	No gaps in refill	q visit													
Technique	Patient inhaler demonstration	Appr. technique	q visit													
Education	Patient/parent understanding	understanding	q visit													
Vaccine	Influenza vaccine	vaccine q fall	q fall													

© 2000, American Society of Health-System Pharmacists, Inc. All rights reserved.

Ambulatory Pharmacist's Care Plan

Patient: Marie Cowling   Pharmacist: Jim Bellows   Date: July 8, 1999

DATE IDENTIFIED	PROBLEM (TPL)	PHARMACOTHERAPEUTIC AND RELATED HEALTH CARE GOAL	RECOMMENDATIONS FOR THERAPY	MONITORING PARAMETER(S)	DESIRED ENDPOINT(S)	MONITORING FREQUENCY
7/8/99	Overuse of Beta-adrenergic agonist	Use Beta-adrenergic agonist appropriately & have good disease control	Add Aerobid 2 puffs BID ↓ use of Maxair use PRN			
	No local health care provider	Establish relationship with local physician	Refer to Joan Owens-social worker for MD Referral			
	No PEF monitoring	PEF monitoring	Daily PEF to establish personal best then periodic assessment			
	Possible drug-disease interaction	No drug-disease interaction	DC ibuprofen use Tylenol for osteoarthritis pain			
	improved disease control	Asthma control	patient education Identify trigger patient will need symptom diary			
	Arthritis	control of arthritis symptoms	DC ibuprofen use Tylenol for osteoarthritis pain			

© 2000, American Society of Health-System Pharmacists, Inc. All rights reserved.

PHARMACIST'S CARE PLAN AMBULATORY MONITORING WORKSHEET (AMW)

Patient _____   Pharmacist _____
                         Date _____

Pharmaco-therapeutic Goal	Monitoring Parameter	Desired Endpoint	Monitoring Frequency	Date												

© 2000, American Society of Health-System Pharmacists, Inc. All rights reserved.

Ambulatory Pharmacist's Care Plan

Patient: Marie Cowling Pharmacist: Jim Bellows Date: July 8, 1999

DATE IDENTIFIED	PROBLEM (TPL)	PHARMACOTHERAPEUTIC AND RELATED HEALTH CARE GOAL	RECOMMENDATIONS FOR THERAPY	MONITORING PARAMETER(S)	DESIRED ENDPOINT(S)	MONITORING FREQUENCY
7/8/99	Overuse of Beta-adrenergic agonist	Use Beta-adrenergic agonist appropriately & have good disease control	Add Aerobid 2 puffs BID ↓ use of Maxair use PRN	Patient report Refill hx	Appropriate use of beta-adrenergic agonist	each visit
	No local health care provider	Establish relationship with local physician	Refer to Joan Owens–social worker for MD Referral	√ c̄ patient	patient establishes relationship with local provider	N/A
	No PEF monitoring	PEF monitoring	Daily PEF to establish personal best then periodic assessment	Patient diary	patient able to self-manage symptoms	each visit
	Possible drug-disease interaction	No drug-disease interaction	DC ibuprofen use Tylenol for osteoarthritis pain	Patient report	relief from arthritis	each visit
	improved disease control	Asthma control	patient education identify trigger patient will need symptom diary	Patient report ↑ Qa–walking c̄/o sx	symptom control	each visit
	Arthritis	control of arthritis symptoms	DC ibuprofen use Tylenol for osteoarthritis pain	Patient report	Relief from arthritis	each visit

© 2000, American Society of Health-System Pharmacists, Inc. All rights reserved.

PHARMACIST'S CARE PLAN AMBULATORY MONITORING WORKSHEET (AMW)

Patient **Marie Cowling**
Pharmacist **Jim Bellows**
Date **July 1999**

Pharmaco-therapeutic Goal	Monitoring Parameter	Desired Endpoint	Monitoring Frequency	Date												
Symptom control	Patient diary	minimal symptoms	pt's daily diary & visit													
PEF monitoring	Patient diary	establish personal best	next visit													
Arthritis control	Patient report	free of symptoms	each visit													
Medication use →	Maxair use	<1 canister per month	each visit													
	AeroBID use	No gaps	each visit													

© 2000, American Society of Health-System Pharmacists, Inc. All rights reserved.

Ambulatory Pharmacist's Care Plan

Patient __Mary Franklin__   Pharmacist __Cheryl Marks__   Date __9/20/99__

DATE IDENTIFIED	PROBLEM (TPL)	PHARMACOTHERAPEUTIC AND RELATED HEALTH CARE GOAL	RECOMMENDATIONS FOR THERAPY	MONITORING PARAMETER(S)	DESIRED ENDPOINT(S)	MONITORING FREQUENCY
9/20/99	Overuse of Beta-adrenergic agonist	Appropriate use & maintain disease control	Evaluate for addition of inhaled corticosteroid			
	No local provider	Local health care provider identified	Given names of physicians			
	No PEF monitoring	Daily PEF reading to establish personal best & periodic	Education			
	Baseline Education	Understanding of medication use and disease	Education			
	Asthma poorly controlled	Education medication management	Add inhaled corticosteroid AeroBid 3 puffs BID			
			Rec Zileuton 20 mg BID			

PHARMACIST'S CARE PLAN AMBULATORY MONITORING WORKSHEET (AMW)

Patient _____   Pharmacist _____
                          Date _____

Pharmaco-therapeutic Goal	Monitoring Parameter	Desired Endpoint	Monitoring Frequency	Date												

© 2000, American Society of Health-System Pharmacists, Inc. All rights reserved.

Part III

Managing an Ambulatory Pharmacist's Care Plan for Patients with Asthma

Implementing a Pharmacist's Care Plan for Patients with Asthma

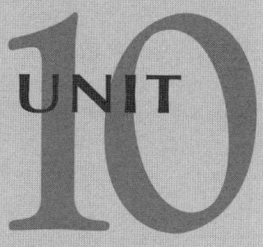
UNIT 10

Unit Objectives	260
Unit Organization	260
Communicating the Plan to Pertinent Health Care Providers	260
Case Study	261
Unique Patient Education Delivery Methods	262
Educational Plan	263
Special Concerns in Continuity of Care	263
Practice Example	263
Summary	264
Reference	264
Self-Study Questions	265
Self-Study Answers	267
Appendix	268

Up to this point in this module, you have learned how to collect data necessary for making therapy decisions, identify pharmacotherapeutic problems, define goals and a therapy regimen, and design a monitoring plan for an ambulatory care patient with asthma. Now you need to implement the plan and assess outcomes of therapy. Therapy adjustments will need to be made along the way.

Unit Objectives

After you successfully complete this unit, you will be able to:
- explain portions of a pharmacist's care plan for an ambulatory care asthma patient that need to be communicated to the pertinent health care providers,
- explain portions of a pharmacist's care plan for an ambulatory care asthma patient that need to be communicated to those outside the health care system who are responsible for ensuring the patient's health,
- explain effective delivery methods unique to patient education programs for ambulatory care patients with asthma,
- formulate an effective plan for the delivery of patient-specific education programs for ambulatory care patients with asthma, and
- explain special concerns in providing continuity of care to patients with asthma.

Unit Organization

This unit begins by reviewing which portions of the ambulatory care pharmacist's care plan need to be communicated to other health care and non–health care providers. Next, we address unique patient education delivery methods. Finally, we discuss continuity-of-care concerns. Practice case studies will be provided.

Unit 17 of the *Core Module* addresses implementation issues. The present unit covers how to communicate your plan with a patient and other health care providers. Throughout this module you have seen examples of pharmacists working collaboratively with patients in the development of care plans. These same principles apply when implementing a plan. The patient needs to be a partner and must share ownership for the plan and its outcomes. Other members of the health care team must understand the goals of pharmacologic therapy.

Communicating the Plan to Pertinent Health Care Providers

In practice sites where you do not have the ability to initiate or modify drug therapy, you must communicate your plan to the responsible health care provider. There is no guarantee that he or she will accept your plan or change a patient's medication regimen. Information that the health care provider shares with you may require that you refine your therapy plan based on new information. Often, negotiation between you and the primary health care provider will take place. The ultimate goal of this negotiation is to reach a compromise that will be beneficial and acceptable to the patient.

Even if you are permitted in your practice setting to modify a patient's therapy, you need to communicate these changes to the patient's primary care provider. Other health care team members should also be informed of any changes that will affect their management of the patient. The means by which this communication is to be accomplished may vary from patient to patient. The type of communication is also mandated by the proximity of your setting to the health care provider's practice site. In some instances, a phone call or personal visit is sufficient. In other cases, a facsimile, e-mail, or letter may be appropriate. These types of communication need to be clarified with each practitioner. If written communication is not used, a follow-up letter should be sent. This documentation will be important for record keeping.

In addition to recommendations for therapy themselves, additional information is important to communicate. Communicate goals that relate to the changes you are suggesting as well as the expected outcome for each medication, in the event that you do not see the patient again. Without these pieces of information, medications are often continued indefinitely. As we have discussed, each medication should be associated with a pharmacotherapeutic or health-related goal.

Case Study

Let's take a look at the case of Jeremy Morgan. Mrs. Morgan's friend suggested that Jeremy's mother seek help from the pharmacist. Fortunately for this pharmacist (Jennifer Loudon), Jeremy's primary care provider, Dr. Lefton, is familiar with her asthma services. Dr. Lefton has many patients that are followed by this pharmacist. Remember that the pharmacist referred Jeremy back to Dr. Lefton because Jeremy had been depending on emergency room visits rather than working more closely with Dr. Lefton. Dr. Lefton already had an understanding and appreciation of the services that this particular pharmacist was able to provide. This understanding on Dr. Lefton's part will make getting recommendations implemented easier. A mutual rapport and respect for each other's knowledge is already in place. A collaborative environment has already been established.

After collecting and reviewing the pertinent data, identifying pharmacotherapy and health-related problems, and developing a list of proposed interventions, the pharmacist prepares to contact Dr. Lefton. As discussed in the *Core Module*, the steps involved in communicating with other health care providers are to:
- present the plan,
- evaluate the provider's response,
- assess/identify issues,
- negotiate the plan, and
- make necessary changes to (i.e., fine tune) the original plan.

Dr. Lefton and Jennifer Loudon frequently have telephone interactions regarding patient therapy plans. Before calling Dr. Lefton, Jennifer contacted her receptionist, set up a time to speak with Dr. Lefton, and faxed a copy of the plan to her office. This gave Dr. Lefton time to review Jeremy's information and prepare herself for the call. More than likely, if Jennifer had not contacted the receptionist and established a time for Dr. Lefton to return the call, Jennifer would have needed to wait for Dr. Lefton to call back when she wasn't in with a patient. Let's listen in on a portion of the phone conversation:

PHARMACIST:
"Dr. Lefton, this is Jennifer from Breathe Rite Pharmacy. I saw Jeremy Morgan the other day. I went ahead and assessed his therapy, but I told him to make an appointment to see you in the next several days. It seems he's had several exacerbations in the past several months and is relying on the emergency room for the majority of his care. As you probably noted from the fax I sent over, I thought we may want to change his therapy a bit."

DR. LEFTON:
"I reviewed your suggestions and appreciate the time you took with Jeremy and his mother. I have had a great deal of difficulty getting Jeremy in the office for a full review of his problems. He's been using the ER more than he has been using me to treat his exacerbations. It is really frustrating. He is coming in to see me tomorrow."

PHARMACIST:
"Great! Why don't I go over what I've come up with and then you can think about my suggestions after you've seen him. If you agree with the changes, just send Jeremy over and I'll fill the prescriptions and go over a treatment and action plan with him."

DR. LEFTON:
"Sounds great! Go ahead and tell me what you've come up with."

PHARMACIST:
"I've counseled Jeremy on his current medications and the importance of taking them. With his nighttime symptoms, I thought we might add Serevent 2 puffs at bedtime. I also thought that switching his current inhaled corticosteroid from Azmacort to Pulmicort might help with adherence, because he'll need to use it only twice a day and it will be also less puffs per day. Do you agree with this plan?"

DR. LEFTON:
"Those sound like good changes to me as long as Jeremy and his mother are willing to try them. Mrs. Morgan has been resistant to corticosteroids for a long time. I knew Jeremy wasn't being adherent. I'll assess Jeremy tomorrow and send him over with any new prescriptions. What about peak flow measurements? Should we have Jeremy check his daily?"

PHARMACIST:
"I think we should try daily peak flow measure-

ments with Jeremy. He doesn't seem to recognize his symptoms. Maybe this will help alert him that he needs to step up his therapy. He has a meter, but hasn't been using it. I've already shown him how to use his meter. His insurance will cover the cost of a spacer, so I'll instruct him on that too. I'll update his action plan and send you a copy for your files. I'll send you an update as soon as I've seen him."

DR. LEFTON:
"Thanks, Jennifer; I appreciate your sending him in to see me. Talk to you soon."

The pharmacist initially met with Jeremy on March 6, 1999. At this time she completed her initial assessment, created her database, and completed medication teaching. Over the next few days, she developed her care plan, sent a copy to Dr. Lefton, and scheduled the telephone appointment with Dr. Lefton. The telephone appointment took place on March 9, 1999. No other health care referrals were needed at this time.

On March 10, 1999, the pharmacist met with Jeremy and his mother to discuss the new prescriptions and review Jeremy's action plan.

PHARMACIST:
"Hi, Jeremy. How are you? Did you bring your mom along? Did you want her to listen in with us today?"

JEREMY:
"Hi. Yeah, my mom is here. She can come in if she wants."

Jeremy, Mrs. Morgan, and the pharmacist go to in the consultation room.

PHARMACIST:
"Jeremy, how have you been feeling? Any difficulty with breathing? Have you needed to use your albuterol inhaler?"

JEREMY:
"Well, I'm still waking up at night coughing and have needed to use my inhaler a couple of times this past week."

PHARMACIST:
"I spoke with Dr. Lefton this week, and we decided to make a few changes in your medications. Maybe we'll be able to stop those nighttime sleep interruptions."

The pharmacist goes over the treatment plan changes and gives Jeremy a written copy of the action plan (**Appendix A**). The pharmacist observed Jeremy demonstrate both his inhaler and peak flow meter, and Jeremy and Mrs. Morgan were given a chance to ask questions. Jeremy and the pharmacist worked out the best times for medication administration and picked times that would be least likely to interfere with his school and social schedule. The pharmacist also gave Jeremy the responsibility of telling his teachers about his asthma when exacerbations occurred. He agreed to give the school nurse a copy of his action plan and said that, if he could really control his symptoms, he would love to run again on the cross-country team this coming fall.

PHARMACIST:
"I think these changes will help you get better control of your asthma. Using this particular inhaled corticosteroid will mean you don't need as many inhalations for each dose. Do you think you will be able to follow this plan, Jeremy? Is the action plan clear to you?"

JEREMY:
"I'm willing to give it a try."

MRS. MORGAN:
"Thanks for all of your help. Does Jeremy need to come and see you again?"

PHARMACIST:
"Yes, I'd like to see Jeremy again in the next few weeks. I'd like to make sure I see Jeremy every month or two for a few months so that we can be sure the changes we have made have improved his asthma control. Jeremy, don't forget, though, that you can come and see me any time you have questions or think you may be having difficulty with your asthma."

Unique Patient Education Delivery Methods

Asthma education requires demonstration and practice of inhaler and peak flow measurement skills. Pharmacists should be able to demonstrate appropriate use of these devices and encourage patients to demonstrate skills at each appointment. Correct peak flow technique was discussed in unit 2. A patient education piece that provides instruction on inhaler technique can be found in unit 8. These activities are best accomplished through individual education sessions. Personal attention allows patients to have hands-on practice under the supervision of a knowledgeable professional.

Color coding action plans into a green zone (all clear), yellow zone (caution), and red zone (medical alert) is a unique way of teaching patients how to react to their asthma based on symptoms outlined in each zone. An example action plan can be found in Appendix A. In some cases, marking zones in color on the peak flow meter may provide a visual reminder for the patient. Action plans are also best reinforced on an individual basis. The concepts and need for a general action plan could be reinforced in a group setting; however, individual parameters should be privately reviewed.

When educating a patient about the action of each medication, identifying the medication as a reliever or controller may be helpful for the patient. A patient may better remember prophylactic medications, such as anti-inflammatory agents, as controller medications. Medications used to treat acute symptoms and provide quick relief are reliever medications. This type of analogy may be especially beneficial in young patients and patients having a difficult time distinguishing the use of each medication.

Group education sessions and support groups can be useful to provide general information about medications and an asthma overview. A group session can be useful because there is usually one person in each group who will begin to ask questions. These questions and their answers may stimulate additional questions that patients had been reluctant to ask. Also, the experiences shared by individuals in the group can reinforce many of the concepts you are trying to convey.

Regardless of whether the session is personal or group, patients should always be given a brief written summary of the information to take with them.

Educational Plan

Educational efforts should not be consolidated into a single, in-depth educational session. Instead, efforts should be broken into manageable portions that will give patients enough information without overwhelming them. For example, a patient newly diagnosed with asthma will need education about disease, triggers, medications, and action plans. Trying to provide all of this information in one session would be overwhelming for a patient. Instead, you might spend the first two sessions covering the disease itself. The next session might focus on the medications used to treat asthma. The following sessions might include a review of known triggers and development of an action plan. With each session, a review of previously covered material is also important. The amount of material that should be covered with each session will vary depending on the patient's available time, motivation, learning style, and interest. Many of the concepts will need to be reinforced over long periods of time. As you get to know the patient and his or her learning style, additional venues other than one-on-one sessions can be worked into the educational plan.

Special Concerns in Continuity of Care

Because asthma can be variable and episodic in nature, continuity of care is essential to the overall care of the patient. Patients, like Jeremy, who have poorly controlled asthma and regularly use the services of emergency rooms and urgent care centers will have gaps in their continuity of care if these visits are not reported to the primary health care provider. With lapses in continuity like these, it will be difficult for a health care provider to accurately assess a patient's overall health and disease control.

Unit 17 in the *Core Module* provides several examples that can be used to facilitate continuity of care in ambulatory care patients. Patients who need follow-up care can have their future visits scheduled before they leave your office. Reminder calls regarding appointments are also helpful for maintaining continuity of care. During calls, ask patients if they have any questions about their medications or disease. Asking patients questions when they are at home and have had time to reflect on previous discussions may trigger further thoughts or questions that were missed during the face-to-face interaction.

Practice Example

Let's return to Mr. Kelley. His information can be found in unit 7, Appendix C. How will the pharmacist maintain continuity of care with Mr. Kelley? Jot down your response, and, when you've finished, compare your answers to what is written below.

The pharmacist initially approached Mr. Kelley about his need for an over-the-counter inhaler. The pharmacist then referred Mr. Kelley to his primary care provider. Following that visit, Mr. Kelley came to see the pharmacist. The initial interaction took place on May 2, 1999. Mr. Kelley returned to the pharmacy on May 5, 1999. He brought all of the information the physician gave with him, including a physical exam report. The pharmacist reviewed asthma management, medication use, and peak flow monitoring with Mr. Kelley at that time. The pharmacist developed a therapeutic plan for Mr. Kelley following his visit on May 5th. The only major referral Mr. Kelley needed was to social services, for financial help due to his lack of a prescription drug benefit. The pharmacist also made the following notations on his follow-up plan for Mr. Kelley:

- Evaluate possible resources to help with payment for medications for Mr. Kelley: social services referral; pharmacist will look into manufacturer reimbursement programs. Referral letter sent to social worker.
- Medication just initiated: will see patient again in one month to assess therapy and response.
- Patient given information about local American Lung Association support groups. Mr. Kelley indicated interest.
- Patient has history of hypertension; no organized exercise program. Patient to check with physician regarding regular exercise program. Pharmacist will need to ascertain the answer to this question during follow-up appointments.

The pharmacist made a note to place a reminder call to Mr. Kelley about his next appointment on June 12, 1999.

Summary

Once you have designed a therapy regimen, you must implement it. Uses of the telephone, in-person visit, facsimile, or e-mail are possible modes of communication. Remember to follow up with patients regarding medications, therapy plans, referrals and any other issues that arise. Documentation of all patient and health care provider interactions will be necessary for assuring continuity of care.

Reference

1. National Heart, Lung, and Blood Institute. Expert Panel Report 2: Guidelines for the Diagnosis and Management of Asthma. July 1997.

Self-Study Questions

Objective
Explain portions of a pharmacist's care plan for an ambulatory care asthma patient that need to be communicated to the pertinent health care providers.

1. Name and explain portions of a pharmacist's care plan for an ambulatory care asthma patient that need to be communicated to the patient's pertinent health care provider.

2. Explain why medication changes need to be communicated to the patient's pertinent health care providers.

3. Explain why treatment goals need to be communicated to the patient's pertinent health care providers.

Objective
Explain portions of a pharmacist's care plan for an ambulatory care asthma patient that need to be communicated to those outside the health care system who are responsible for ensuring the patient's health.

Refer to the case of Marie Cowling.

4. Explain why the action plan needs to be communicated to Marie.

Refer to the case of Jeremy Morgan (Appendix A).

5. Explain why Jeremy's coaches need to be familiar with Jeremy's action plan.

6. Consider Josie, a 4-year-old girl with moderate-persistent asthma who is in a day care environment. Explain why her day care provider needs to be familiar with her action plan.

Objective
Explain effective delivery methods unique to patient education programs for ambulatory care patients with asthma.

7. Explain effective delivery methods unique to patient education programs for patients with asthma.

8. Personal or group educational sessions should be followed up with which of the following?
    A. A thank-you letter to promote positive customer relations with the pharmacy department.
    B. A written summary of the material presented in the session.
    C. An assessment of patient satisfaction with the session.
    D. An audiotape of the session.

9. Which of the following educational techniques is most essential for patient education about inhaler and peak flow measurement skills?
    A. written step-by-step instructions with diagrams
    B. videos demonstrating proper techniques
    C. one-on-one demonstration and practice sessions
    D. group lectures

Objective
Formulate an effective plan for the delivery of patient-specific education programs for ambulatory care patients with asthma.

10. Describe a plan for the effective delivery of patient-specific education programs for ambulatory care patients with asthma.

11. Tim is a shy 15-year-old with moderate-persistent asthma. His mother has never pushed his participation in asthma education classes because he is so shy. She says the only time he is really animated is when he is online, chatting. What kind of educational strategies might you use to communicate effectively with Tim?

12. Jane Frye is a corporate attorney for a large international corporation. She spends much of her time traveling from one manufacturing facility to another and is on the road at least 50% of her time. She is also the mother of two grade-school boys. She has recently been diagnosed with asthma. What kind of educational strategies might you use with Jane?

Self-Study Questions (cont.)

Objective
Explain special concerns in providing continuity of care to patients with asthma.

13. Explain special concerns in providing continuity of care to ambulatory care patients with asthma.

14. Explain why emergency room visits are a special concern in providing continuity of care to ambulatory care patients with asthma.

15. Explain why reminder calls may be useful in providing continuity of care to ambulatory care patients with asthma.

Self-Study Answers

1. Recommendations for therapy modification or actual changes that have been made; treatment goals and expected outcomes

2. Therapy changes need to be communicated to other health care professionals so that the other members of the health care team can better evaluate the patient during their next patient-provider encounter.

3. Treatment goals need to be communicated so that other health care professionals can evaluate whether the medication is meeting the stated goal.

4. Marie needs to understand the role of her medications and learn self-management of symptoms.

5. Jeremy's coaches need to understand the action plan that has been developed for Jeremy so that they can make decisions that are in concert with those made by Jeremy and his health care team; also, they must not be either too cavalier or too cautious with their approach to Jeremy and his asthma.

6. It is important for Josie's caregivers to have knowledge of her action plan. There may be times when they will need to implement an increase in her rescue therapy. Without this knowledge, they might either let the episode go too long without treatment or have the parents leave work more frequently than would otherwise be necessary.

7. Education in the use of inhalers, spacers, and peak flow monitoring are best accomplished through one-on-one sessions. Basic asthma education information can be accomplished in a group setting and followed up with a written plan.

8. B

9. C

10. Educational efforts should be broken up in to manageable portions. The amount of information appropriate for each session will be patient dependent.

11. Tim is computer literate and has access to a computer. Using electronic interactive learning tools would probably be more effective than a group session for his learning style. Familiarizing him with available asthma-specific information he can find on the Internet might be useful for him. You might even consider having him track his peak flow readings on a computer rather than by hand.

12. Jane will probably appreciate the environment of a group educational session. She will probably only have the time to attend one or two sessions. Providing her with written information that she can keep with her and read in her available time during travel might be a good option. Coupling this with brief telephone follow-ups for questions that occur will provide Jane with support and efficiency which she will appreciate.

13. Frequent emergency room visits and reminder calls can be special concerns in the ambulatory care patient with asthma.

14. Frequent emergency room visits can result in gaps in continuity of care if these visits are not reported back to the primary health care provider. This can make it difficult for a health care provider to accurately assess a patient's overall health and disease control.

15. Reminder calls can be useful for ambulatory care patients with asthma, not only to remind them to keep needed appointments, but also to serve as a time to ask about problems with or questions about medications or disease control.

ASTHMA ACTION PLAN (EXAMPLE 1)

Name __Jeremy Morgan__ Date __March 10, 1999__

It is important in managing asthma to keep track of your symptoms, medications, and Peak Expiratory Flow (PEF). You can use the colors of a traffic light to help learn your asthma medications:

- A. **GREEN means Go** — Use preventive (anti-inflammatory) medicine.
- B. **YELLOW means Caution** — Use quick-relief (short-acting bronchodilator) medicine in addition to the preventive medicine.
- C. **RED means STOP!** — Get help from a doctor.

A. Your **GREEN ZONE** is __340-425 L/min__ 80 to 100% of your personal best. **GO!**
Breathing is good, with no cough, wheeze, or chest tightness during work, school, exercise, or play.

ACTION:
- ☐ Continue with medications listed in your daily treatment plan.

B. Your **YELLOW ZONE** is __210-340 L/min__ 50 to less than 80% of your personal best. **CAUTION!**
Asthma symptoms are present (cough, wheeze, chest tightness).
Your peak flow number drops below __300 L/min__ or you notice: (for more than 1 reading)
- ☐ Increased need for inhaled quick-relief medicine
- ☐ Increased asthma symptoms upon awakening
- ☐ Awakening at night with asthma symptoms
- ☐ __Difficulty participating in physical activities__

ACTIONS:
- ☐ Take __2__ puffs of your quick-relief (bronchodilator) medicine __Proventil (Albuterol)__ Repeat __1__ times.
- ☐ Take __2__ puffs of __Pulmicort (Budesonide)__ (anti-inflammatory) __2__ times/day.
- ☐ Begin/increase treatment with oral steroids. __call Dr. Lefton's office, do not start on own__
- ☐ Take ____ mg of _____ every a.m. p.m.
- ☐ Call your doctor (phone) __222-3111__ or emergency room __911__

C. Your **RED ZONE** is __210 L/min__ 50% or less of your personal best. **DANGER!!**
Your peak flow number drops below __210 L/min__ or you continue to get worse after increasing treatment according to the directions above.

ACTIONS:
- ☐ Take __2__ puffs of your quick-relief (bronchodilator) medicine __Proventil (Albuterol)__ Repeat __0__ times.
- ☐ Begin/increase treatment with oral steroids. Take ____ mg now.
- ☐ Call your doctor now (phone __222-3111__). If you cannot contact your doctor, go directly to the emergency room (phone __911__).
- ☐ Other important phone numbers for transportation _____ .

AT ANY TIME, CALL YOUR DOCTOR IF:
- ☐ Asthma symptoms worsen while you are taking oral steroids, or
- ☐ Inhaled bronchodilator treatments are not lasting 4 hours, or
- ☐ Your peak flow number remains or falls below __300 L/min__ in spite of following the plan.

Physician Signature __Janet Lefton M.D.__ Patient/Family Member's Signature __Jeremy Morgan__

This plan is provided as an example to clinicians.

Evaluating Outcomes for Patients with Asthma

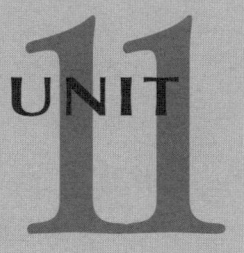

UNIT 11

Unit Objectives 270
Unit Organization 270
Interpreting Monitoring Data 270
Assessing Goal Achievement—Case Study 270
    Patient Status, Condition, and Therapy Changes 270
    Missing Data 271
    Need for Further Data 271
    Achievement of Desired Endpoints 271
    Analyzing Trends 272
    Patient-Specific Education Assessment 272
Practice Example 272
Summary 273
Self-Study Questions 274
Self-Study Answers 275
Appendixes 276

In unit 9, we discussed monitoring parameters necessary to follow in the care of ambulatory care patients with asthma. The next step is to track a patient's progress and evaluate outcomes to determine whether the desired endpoints have been met. You will need to refer back to the AMW and APCP as you assess patient outcomes. The patient will do the bulk of asthma management. This self-management makes it imperative that patient education is continually reinforced and its effectiveness is assessed.

Unit Objectives

After you successfully complete this unit, you will be able to:
- interpret data unique to ambulatory patients with asthma that are gathered as specified in a monitoring plan,
- assess data to determine achievement of or state of progress toward achievement of an ambulatory asthma patient's pharmacotherapeutic and related health care goals,
- determine reasons for an ambulatory asthma patient's progress or lack of progress toward stated health care goals,
- explain the importance of analysis of trends that are unique to the monitoring parameter measurements for ambulatory patients with asthma, and
- assess the effectiveness of patient-specific education programs for ambulatory patients with asthma.

Unit Organization

In this unit, we will discuss and practice the approach to evaluating outcomes, beginning with interpretation of patient monitoring data. This includes the assessment of patient status over time, exacerbations, quality of life, and changes in therapy as well as the review of data needed for a complete evaluation. Next, we will assess the effectiveness of patient-specific education. The case of Jeremy Morgan will be used as a model for evaluating patient outcomes. A practice case (that of Sarah Jacobs) is provided at the end of this unit.

Interpreting Monitoring Data

As you use the patient-specific AMW to evaluate achievement of outcomes, you will need to look at the items listed on the AMW in light of the APCP for each patient. To determine whether the patient has met specified goals, you need to look at the information you have collected on the AMW and evaluate whether:
- you are missing any information,
- there are inconsistencies in the information,
- all the information makes good clinical sense, and
- the information collected is reliable and valid.

Review unit 19 of the *Core Module*, which provides background that will be useful as you use data to evaluate progress towards stated goals.

Assessing Goal Achievement—Case Study

As you begin assessing goal achievement, keep in mind the four steps necessary in this process, covered in more detail in unit 20 of the *Core Module*:
- Consider any changes in patient status, condition, or drug or nondrug therapy since the original AMW plan was developed.
- Assess information for missing data.
- Assess the need for additional data.
- Assess achievement of the desired endpoint for each parameter in the monitoring plan and make a judgement as to whether the pharmacotherapeutic goal was met.

Patient Status, Condition, and Therapy Changes

As you evaluate a patient, include an assessment of changes in the patient's status or condition. Remember that asthma is a highly variable disease. Patients can move quickly from one level of severity to another. Patients considered to have mild-intermittent asthma at an initial visit may easily move to moderate-persistent asthma by the time of the next evaluation (or vice versa). Your goals must be flexible, depending on the patient's overall condition. These changes in status may stem from a multitude of factors, including:

- adherence issues,
- weather changes,
- concurrent diseases,
- new drug therapy (prescription and nonprescription),
- environmental changes,
- psychosocial issues, and
- changes in physical activity.

In the past several months Jeremy Morgan's disease status has been in flux. The pharmacist met with Jeremy on several occasions: March 6, 1999; March 10, 1999; April 3, 1999; May 5, 1999; June 20, 1999; and July 30, 1999. Changes in Jeremy's pharmacotherapy were not implemented until the second appointment. Springtime tends to aggravate Jeremy's asthma and he required a step up in therapy during the last part of April and May. He suffered one exacerbation that required an urgent care visit in May. Since that time, he was able to step down his therapy and (by self-report) has been relatively adherent with his medication administration and peak flow monitoring. The severity of his asthma was recorded as mild-persistent during his last evaluation. This was quite a change from his initial visit. The pharmacist will not be able to evaluate the effect of Jeremy's participation in the cross-country track team will have on his asthma until school starts up again in the fall. By helping Jeremy manage his asthma and encouraging him to join the team, he may very well meet that goal. Your goals on the AMW and APCP (**Appendix A**) should still be current for Jeremy at this time.

Remember to keep these changes in mind as you evaluate your patient. Some patients may develop concurrent diseases that necessitate new drug therapy or may decide to add an herbal medication to their regimen. Failure to take these changes into consideration could provide you with an inaccurate analysis of your patient and may cause you to make inappropriate recommendations.

Missing Data

An evaluation of the AMW will alert you to missing data. In Jeremy's case, very little data is required. You measure a peak flow with each appointment. Jeremy keeps a daily log at home and records his PEF. You have asked him to bring this in with his appointments, but he continually forgets. Although this information is not essential to his evaluation, it would help identify trends. The pharmacist should consider calling Jeremy before his next appointment to remind him to bring in the log. Use caution with this data because it is a patient self-report. Some patients are not adherent with self-monitoring and may simply record numbers in the log. Keep this in mind as you evaluate the reliability of self-reported information.

Patients may require other forms of monitoring, such as PFTs, serum drug concentrations, and LFTs. Make sure you receive this information to use in your evaluation. This information can help you assess trends in asthma control and evaluate potential adverse drug effects.

Need for Further Data

You will need to continually evaluate your patient's changing status to determine whether additional data is required. Potential sources of additional data may stem from changes to the patient's medication regimen or a referral to a specialist. If a patient sees a new health care provider, you will want to make sure that your goals are still in line with those of both the patient and the other health care providers. Patient goals may change over time. You must readdress goals on an ongoing basis.

Achievement of Desired Endpoints

As you assess the achievement of desired endpoints for each parameter in the monitoring plan, you will need to decide whether the defined pharmacotherapeutic goal was met. You will also want to make sure that the desired endpoints continue to be valid for your patient. If the endpoints are valid and an endpoint has not been met, you must determine reasons for the lack of progress towards the goal. In the case of asthma, several factors may result in nonachievement of goals. Adherence is certainly one factor to consider, as well as whether life changes have occurred for a patient that are adding barriers to his or her therapy. Is the patient experiencing a new stress in his or her life? Remember the case of Molly introduced in unit 7. The break up of Molly's parents' marriage was impacting her asthma management. Changes in weather, environmental factors, job, school, home, physical health, and social activities may all contribute to a lack of goal achievement. In some cases, a medication and monitoring regimen that was once manageable becomes overwhelming in the midst of daily life. You will need to carefully dig down and find the underlying reason for a lack of progress. Keep in mind that the nature of asthma is variable and so, too, must the therapeutic plan be. Viewing a plan as dynamic in nature allows you and the patient to alter the plan as needed and to continually assess its appropriateness.

Analyzing Trends

As you evaluate the achievement of outcomes, you should analyze trends rather than values from single points in time. In addition, you need to analyze the most recent peak flow measurements and symptom management. In Jeremy's case (Appendix A), by analyzing trends, you are able to determine that even though he had increased symptoms in the springtime, his overall ability to control symptoms and prevent ER visits has improved dramatically. It is important to continue to monitor Jeremy's disease management because school and cross-country track will be starting and his ability to remain motivated may deteriorate.

Let's look a little closer at the case of Jeremy. At his last visit (September 20, 1999, following the start of school) the pharmacist was finally able to get Jeremy to bring his peak flow monitoring diary along with him for his appointment. On looking over the diary for the past several weeks, it appeared that Jeremy was experiencing a reduction in peak flow measurement Monday through Thursday evenings. This was puzzling to both Jeremy and the pharmacist, especially since Jeremy hadn't noted any worsening symptoms. He also had made a decision not to step up his therapy because it would interfere with his school schedule. On further discussion, they both realized that these were the days that Jeremy had cross-country track practice in both the afternoon and the evening. By looking at the trend, they identified a need to re-evaluate Jeremy's current regimen before his asthma symptoms interfered with his ability to participate on the team.

Patient-Specific Education Assessment

As discussed in previous units and the *Core Module*, education programs are an important component of any patient plan. Unit 8 provides a discussion of the necessary components of an education plan. As you assess the impact of your educational efforts on each patient, you will want to be able to track the patient's progress. The best way to do this is to determine objectives for each educational topic, document what was taught and the patient's understanding, and evaluate the outcome for that objective. In Jeremy's case, the pharmacist determined that the most critical education component was the need to understand the seriousness of asthma and appropriate symptom management. His educational plan included these goals:

- describe the airways of a patient with asthma,
- state the potential consequences of uncontrolled asthma,
- state triggers and actions that need to be taken when exposures or exacerbations are noted, and
- demonstrate inhaler and peak flow monitoring technique.

As each item in this plan is taught, the pharmacist should note the date taught and the patient's level of understanding (e.g., "achieved outcome," "requires assistance," "needs further education," or "declines instruction"). This documentation will provide the pharmacist with a record of what has been taught and what requires further attention. Certain items will need to be continually reinforced with each visit, while others may simply be assessed periodically. Education should be incorporated into every session with a patient.

Practice Example

Turn now to the case of Sarah Jacobs (**Appendix B**). We first introduced Sarah in unit 8. Sarah is a 4-year-old child newly diagnosed with asthma. She was initially seen in the clinic in April. Her physician prescribed nedocromil and albuterol for management of her disease. Her educational needs included: education of child and parents on basics of asthma, medication use and role, environmental control, and daily symptom management; inhaler technique; symptom recognition; and skills.

Review Sarah's AMW and determine the reliability of the data. Has Sarah achieved her goals? Is she making progress towards these goals? If not, what are the reasons she is not reaching these goals? What types of questions would you ask to assess the effectiveness of education provided to Sarah and her family?

The first step in the assessment is to determine whether there have been any changes in the patient's status or condition. Were changes to drug therapy made? In this case, Sarah had two ER visits in December, but no changes in her therapy were made. Peak flow monitoring was not initiated, so the only parameter you have to assess from this patient other than exacerbations requiring urgent or emergent care is her need to use rescue therapy. Her need for albuterol increased in December, but leveled off the first 2 weeks of January.

Your next step is to assess and evaluate achievement of desired endpoints. Sarah's first health care goal was control of her asthma. Quite obviously, she has not achieved this goal as evidenced by her ER visits in December. You need to determine the factors causing these ER visits. Is therapy inadequate? Was the patient exposed to a trigger? Is there a compliance issue? On talking with Sarah's mother, you discover that both ER visits occurred during the holidays. The first visit happened while Sarah was visiting her father. Her father was confused about the medications and forgot to give them to Sarah for a couple of days. Sarah was sick with a chest cold at the time and the lack of medications resulted in an exacerbation, and she required oral prednisone for 5 days. The second ER visit occurred 10 days after the previous one, when Sarah was visiting relatives. Sarah's mother, thinking that a couple of missed doses wouldn't create a problem, forgot to include Sarah's medicine with her bags. Unfortunately, the relatives had many pets, and Sarah again needed an ER visit.

Sarah demonstrates an inhaler technique that varies with each demonstration.

Now that the holidays are over, everything seems back to normal and Sarah is doing fine. Therefore, it appears that over a long period of time there is a trend towards adherence with therapy and good symptom control. The holidays brought about a few changes that resulted in nonadherence. Reinforcement of education should be targeted at these points. Both Sarah and her parents (as well as other caregivers) need to understand the seriousness of asthma and receive education regarding symptom management and the importance of adherence.

Summary

Assessing the status of desired endpoints for selected parameters provides the pharmacist with a framework for determining whether goals have successfully been achieved. Using a systematic approach to this assessment helps eliminate confusion and inadvertent omission of information. Before an adjustment is made to the APCP, the pharmacist should determine the cause of failure to attain the therapeutic goals.

Self-Study Questions

Objective
Interpret data unique to ambulatory patients with asthma that are gathered as specified in a monitoring plan.

Refer to the case of Marie Cowling (**Appendix C**). Interpret her monitoring data.

1. Which data would you assess to determine whether Ms. Cowling's health care goal of good asthma control has been achieved?

2. Which data would you assess to determine whether Ms. Cowling's health care goal of arthritis control has been achieved?

3. Which data would you assess to determine whether Ms. Cowling has achieved her goal of PEF monitoring?

Objective
Assess data to determine achievement of or state of progress toward achievement of an ambulatory asthma patient's pharmacotherapeutic and related health care goals.

Refer to the case of Marie Cowling (Appendix C).

4. What do the PEF measurements indicate about this patient's progress toward her goals?

5. What does the patient's report of asthma symptom frequency indicate about her progress towards her goals?

6. What does the patient's refill history for Maxair indicate about her progress towards her goals?

Objective
Determine reasons for an ambulatory asthma patient's progress or lack of progress towards stated health care goals.

7. Give a reason why Ms. Cowling has not achieved good control of her asthma symptoms.

8. Give a reason why Ms. Cowling has not achieved her goal of monitoring peak flow.

9. Give a reason why Ms. Cowling has not achieved her goal of improved quality of life, which is walking without developing an asthma exacerbation.

Objective
Explain the importance of analysis of trends that are unique to the monitoring parameter measurements for ambulatory patients with asthma.

10. Explain the importance of the analysis of trends that are unique to the monitoring parameter measurements of ambulatory care patients with asthma.

11. Which of the following is an example of important information that may be discovered when analyzing trends for an ambulatory care asthma patient?
    A. relevant information about the patient's work habits
    B. the patient's vacation schedule
    C. the type of people the patient associates with
    D. increased exacerbations during certain seasons of the year

12. Which of the following best describes why information learned when analyzing trends may be important?
    A. It is a good teaching tool for other members of the health care team.
    B. Plans can be made to handle times when exacerbations are found to be higher.
    C. It can provide evidence for the need for increased funding in the pharmacy.
    D. Trends for one patient can be generalized to other patients.

Objective
Assess the effectiveness of patient-specific education programs for ambulatory patients with asthma.

Refer to the case of Marie Cowling.

13. How would you assess the effectiveness of patient-specific information for this patient?

Self-Study Answers

1. patient report of symptoms, refill history, and peak flow self-monitoring results
2. patient report
3. peak flow self-monitoring diary and patient demonstration of technique
4. Patient has not measured PEF; cannot use as an assessment.
5. Patient continues with frequent symptoms; not progressing.
6. Patient continues to use Maxair excessively.
7. patient may have an unidentified trigger for exacerbations; patient may need to use a holding chamber because of difficulty with inhaler coordination from arthritis; adherence to inhaled corticosteroid may be an issue.
8. Patient refuses to monitor peak flow.
9. Patient's asthma continues to be poorly controlled.
10. It is important to assess trends in symptom exacerbation, adherence, adverse effects, and peak flow measurement. These trends may identify particular triggers for a patient or identify factors that are affecting appropriate disease control.
11. D
12. B
13. You should ask the patient questions about the underlying cause of asthma, monitoring parameters, symptom recognition, action plan, and disease progression. You should have the patient demonstrate inhaler and peak flow monitoring technique.

Ambulatory Pharmacist's Care Plan

Patient **Jeremy Morgan** Pharmacist **Jennifer Loudon** Date **March 10, 1999**

DATE IDENTIFIED	PROBLEM (TPL)	PHARMACOTHERAPEUTIC AND RELATED HEALTH CARE GOAL	RECOMMENDATIONS FOR THERAPY	MONITORING PARAMETER(S)	DESIRED ENDPOINT(S)	MONITORING FREQUENCY
3/99	overuse of Albuterol	minimize symptoms optimize therapeutic regimen	D/C Neb solution Institute Serevent 2 puffs @ HS	Frequency & severity of nighttime sx; monitor PEF	PEF >80% No morning dip in PEF; No nighttime symptoms	Each visit
	intermittent refill record Azmacort	optimize education & medication administration	Δ to 1 puff BID Pulmicort	PEF Refill hx symptom diary	Normal PEF No exacerbations adherence	Each visit
	cigarette & alcohol use	protect confidentiality while educating about risks	Education	Patient report	No exposure	Each visit
	self-monitoring not done	Add peak flow monitoring	Daily PEF & Diary	Diary evaluation	Daily monitor	Each visit
	poor symptom recognition Echinacea use for prolonged time	Educate about symptoms	Education	Patient report	Recognition of symptoms	Each visit
	Influenza	Discontinue Echinacea	Discontinue	Patient/Parent Report	D/C	Each visit
	Vaccine: Not vaccinated	Vaccinate yearly	Vaccinate in the fall	Patient records	vaccination	Every fall
	Misconceptions about corticosteroids	Provide Education	Education	Patient report adherence	adherence	Each visit

© 2000, American Society of Health-System Pharmacists, Inc. All rights reserved.

PHARMACIST'S CARE PLAN AMBULATORY MONITORING WORKSHEET (AMW)

Patient _Jeremy Morgan_   Pharmacist _Jennifer Loudon_
                           Date _3/4/99_

Pharmaco-therapeutic Goal	Monitoring Parameter	Desired Endpoint	Monitoring Frequency	3/10/99	4/3	5/5	6/20	7/30	9/20
Improve asthma control	Symptom Diary	↓ freq. of sx	q month		↑sx ✓	↑sx ✓	↓sx ✓	↓sx ✓	↓sx ✓
	(refill hx) Beta-adrenergic agonist use	<1 canister per month	q month		OK	OK	OK	OK	OK
	(refill hx) Pulmicort use	No gaps in refill	q month		OK	OK	OK	OK	OK
↓	Nighttime Sx	None	(patient) Daily		←	ER visit ↑	→	→	←
Monitoring of peak flow	Morning PEF	Daily ✓'s	(patient) Daily		420	400	420	420	420
	Influenza vaccine	Given	q fall		–	–	–	–	done
Education	Patient knowledge	Understanding	q visit		✓	✓	✓	✓	✓
	Inhaler technique	Appropriate	q visit		✓	✓	✓	✓	✓
↓ Monitoring	Evening PEF	Daily ✓'s	q visit		started ✓'s	440 ✓	450 ✓	450 ✓	390 ↓
Cigarette & alcohol education	Patient/parent report	0 exposures	q visit		2-3	5	1	2	2
d/c echinacea	Patient/parent report	D/C	q visit		Patient is still using				

© 2000, American Society of Health-System Pharmacists, Inc. All rights reserved.

Ambulatory Pharmacist's Care Plan

Patient: Sarah Jacobs Pharmacist: Bill Jelen Date: 4-99

DATE IDENTIFIED	PROBLEM (TPL)	PHARMACOTHERAPEUTIC AND RELATED HEALTH CARE GOAL	RECOMMENDATIONS FOR THERAPY	MONITORING PARAMETER(S)	DESIRED ENDPOINT(S)	MONITORING FREQUENCY
4/6/99	New diagnosis asthma-associated w/viral illness	control of sxs	Tilade 2 puffs qid Albuterol qid prn	symptoms exacerbations refill hx gaps in refill	minimal sxs no exacerbations, appropriate refills	q visit q refill
4/6	Basic asthma education needed	Education	Set up education plan—will need to include both parents	✓ patient/parent understanding	patient/parent understanding pathophys & meds	q visit
4/6	No flu vaccine	vaccination in fall	schedule in fall	✓ if received	vaccinated	q fall

*12/99 received oral prednisone X 5 days exac resulted from exp to resp virus, failure to adhere to tx regimen

© 2000, American Society of Health-System Pharmacists, Inc. All rights reserved.

PHARMACIST'S CARE PLAN AMBULATORY MONITORING WORKSHEET (AMW)

Patient __Sarah Jacobs__   Pharmacist __Bill Jelen__
                            Date __4-6-99__

Pharmaco-therapeutic Goal	Monitoring Parameter	Desired Endpoint	Monitoring Frequency	Date 4/6	5/20	6/30	9/30	11/20	1/20							
Asthma control	Symptom diary	No symptoms	q visit		OK ✓	OK ✓	OK ✓	OK ✓	x2 ER visits c/d sxs							
Med adherence	Albuterol refill hx	<1 cannister per month	q visit		✓	*	*	*	*							
Med adherence	Tilade refill hx	No gaps in refill	q visit		✓	*	*	*	*							
Technique	Patient inhaler demonstration	Appr. technique	q visit		some difficulty	improved	good	not as good	poor							
Education	Patient/parent understanding	Understanding	q visit		needs help	improved	improved	good	good							
Vaccine	Influenza vaccine	Vaccine q fall	q fall		—	—	vaccinated	—	—							

*cannot evaluate due to medications filled @ multiple pharmacies

© 2000, American Society of Health-System Pharmacists, Inc. All rights reserved.

Ambulatory Pharmacist's Care Plan

Patient: Marie Cowling Pharmacist: Jim Bellows Date: July 8, 1999

DATE IDENTIFIED	PROBLEM (TPL)	PHARMACOTHERAPEUTIC AND RELATED HEALTH CARE GOAL	RECOMMENDATIONS FOR THERAPY	MONITORING PARAMETER(S)	DESIRED ENDPOINT(S)	MONITORING FREQUENCY
7/8/99	Overuse of Beta-adrenergic agonist	Use Beta-adrenergic agonist appropriately & have good disease control	Add Aerobid 2 puffs BID, ↓ use of Maxair use PRN	Patient report Refill hx	Appropriate use of beta-adrenergic agonist	each visit
	No local health care provider	Establish relationship with local physician	Refer to Joan Owens—social worker for MD Referral	√ c̄ patient	patient establishes relationship with local provider	N/A
	No PEF monitoring	PEF monitoring	Daily PEF to establish personal best then periodic assessment	Patient diary	patient able to self-manage symptoms	each visit
	Possible drug-disease interaction	No drug-disease interaction	DC ibuprofen, use Tylenol for osteoarthritis pain	Patient report	relief from arthritis	each visit
	improved disease control	Asthma control	patient education identify trigger patient will need symptom diary	Patient report ↑ Qa-walking c̄/o sx	symptom control	each visit
→	Arthritis	control of arthritis symptoms	DC ibuprofen use Tylenol for osteoarthritis pain	Patient report	Relief from arthritis	each visit

PHARMACIST'S CARE PLAN AMBULATORY MONITORING WORKSHEET (AMW)

Patient: Marie Cowling

Pharmacist: Jim Bellows

Date: July 1999

Pharmaco-therapeutic Goal	Monitoring Parameter	Desired Endpoint	Monitoring Frequency	Date 7/8/99	8/15	9/28	11/20
Symptom control	Patient diary	minimal symptoms	pt ✓'s daily diary q visit		↑ sx	↑ sx	↑ sx
PEF monitoring	Patient diary	establish personal best	next visit		* Re-fuses	* Re-fuses	* Re-fuses
Arthritis control	Patient report	free of symptoms	each visit		↑ sx	↑ sx	↑ sx
medication use →	Maxair use	<1 canister per month	each visit		2 canisters	2 canisters	2 canisters
	AeroBID use	No gaps	each visit		gap in fill	gap in fill	ok

*Pt refuses to monitor PEF

© 2000, American Society of Health-System Pharmacists, Inc. All rights reserved.

Ambulatory Pharmacist's Care Plan

Patient __Mary Franklin__ Pharmacist __Cheryl Marks__ Date __9/20/99__

DATE IDENTIFIED	PROBLEM (TPL)	PHARMACOTHERAPEUTIC AND RELATED HEALTH CARE GOAL	RECOMMENDATIONS FOR THERAPY	MONITORING PARAMETER(S)	DESIRED ENDPOINT(S)	MONITORING FREQUENCY
9/20/99	Overuse of Beta-adrenergic agonist	Appropriate use & maintain disease control	Evaluate for addition of inhaled corticosteroid	Symptom report, symptom diary	Appropriate use	Each visit
	No local provider	Local health care provider identified	Given names of physicians	Patient report	Local health care provider	Next visit
	No PEF monitoring	Daily PEF reading to establish personal best & periodic	Education	Diary	Periodic PEF monitoring	Each visit
	Baseline Education	Understanding of medication use and disease	Education	Patient report	Understanding	Each visit
	Asthma poorly controlled	Education medication management	Add inhaled corticosteroid AeroBid 3 puffs BID	symptoms, PEF, LFTs, refill history	Reduce exacerbations	Each visit, LFTs per protocol
			Rec. zileuton 20mg BID			

* 11/15 Begin zileuton
2/00 Zileuton dc'd ↑AeroBid to 5 puffs BID

© 2000, American Society of Health-System Pharmacists, Inc. All rights reserved.

PHARMACIST'S CARE PLAN AMBULATORY MONITORING WORKSHEET (AMW)

Patient: Mary Franklin
Pharmacist: Patti Belle
Date: Sept. 1999

Pharmaco-therapeutic Goal	Monitoring Parameter	Desired Endpoint	Monitoring Frequency	10/12	11/15	12/15	1/15	2/15	3/15	5/15
Symptom control	pt diary-symptoms	↓ frequency	q visit		←	↓	OK	OK	OK	OK
	Beta-adrenergic agonist (refill hx)	<1 canister/month	q visit		2 canisters	✓	✓	✓	✓	✓
	AeroBid use (refill hx)	No gaps	q visit		gap	OK	OK	OK	OK	OK
	Nighttime sx	No sx	q visit		←	None	None	None	None	None
Monitoring	Morning PEF	daily √'s	q visit		not done	✓ 325	✓ 350	✓ 350	✓ 360	✓ 380
	Influenza vaccine	vaccine	q fall	done						
Knowledge	pt knowledge	understanding	q visit		improving	OK	OK	OK	OK	OK
	Inhaler technique	appropriate	q visit		good	good	good	good	good	good
Adverse effects	ALT	0-35 units/L	q month MD office		5	15	30	60	20	10

© 2000, American Society of Health-System Pharmacists, Inc. All rights reserved.

Assessment of Asthma Self-management Knowledge: Mary Franklin

Completed 2/18/99

Asthma Disease Understanding

1. Describe what happens to the airways in a patient with an asthma exacerbation.

   Mary: "I think your lungs fill with water or fluid or something like that."

Medications

2. State the name of your medication, what it is used for, and when you take it.

   Mary: "I have two inhalers. One is Procardia and the other is AeroBid. I use the AeroBid two times a day. I have to use the Procardia only sometimes when my chest feels tight. I don't know the difference between them."

Monitoring

3. Show me how you use your peak flow meter. What is the purpose of using your peak flow meter?

   (Mary accurately demonstrates peak flow measurement.)
   Mary: "I'm not sure why I measure peak flow other than I was told I should."

Redesigning the Pharmacist's Care Plan for Patients with Asthma

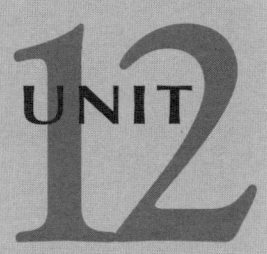

UNIT 12

Unit Objectives	286
Unit Organization	286
Determining the Need for Changes	286
Patient's Quality of Life	286
Change in Patient Status	286
Receipt of Updated or More Complete Patient Information	286
Possible Changes to the Therapy Regimen	287
Adding New Therapy	287
Deleting a Current Therapy	287
Modifying the Current Therapy Regimen	287
Changes in Educational Goals and Plans	287
Change in Therapy	287
Change in Patient Status	288
Stabilization of Patient on Current Therapy	288
Modifying a Pharmacist's Care Plan for Ambulatory Care Patients with Asthma—	
Case Study	288
Goal #1	288
Goal #2	288
Goal #3	288
Goal #4	288
Goal #5	288
Goal #6	289
Goal #7	289
Practice Example	289
Goal #1: Control of Symptoms	289
Goal #2: Education	289
Goal #3: Influenza Vaccine	289
Summary	289
Reference	289
Self-Study Questions	290
Self-Study Answers	291
Appendixes	292

In unit 21 of the *Core Module*, you learned the principles of redesigning the pharmacist's care plan in the ambulatory care setting. Not every plan implemented for a patient will achieve the desired goals. Original plans will need to be continually reviewed and redesigned to meet new goals or to attain the original goals.

Unit Objectives

After you successfully complete this unit, you will be able to:
- determine whether a change in therapeutic and related health care goals, regimen, or monitoring plan is required in the treatment of ambulatory care patients with asthma, and
- modify a pharmacist's care plan for ambulatory care patients with asthma as necessary based on the achievement of pharmacotherapeutic and related health care goals.

Unit Organization

This unit begins with a discussion of how the need for changes in goals, regimen, or monitoring plan of a patient with asthma is determined. Once these needed alterations have been identified, the next section reviews the process of modifying the care plan to reflect these changes.

Determining the Need for Changes

Unit 21 of the *Core Module* discusses three factors that can aid you in identifying whether you need to change your pharmacotherapeutic and related health care goals. These factors are:
- the patient's quality of life,
- change in the patient's status, and
- the receipt of updated or more complete patient information.

Patient's Quality of Life

As discussed in unit 7 of this module, a patient's perception of how disease affects his or her ability to perform the activities of daily living is an important consideration when setting pharmacotherapeutic and related health care goals. Remember that perception of quality of life is subjective. Consider the case of Marie Cowling. She is the retired woman who recently moved to Sun City and has virtually no local support system. We set a goal for her to monitor PEF. Despite our best efforts, Marie refuses to do it. We will have to alter our plan and rely more on her symptom diary, emphasizing in educational sessions the importance of accurate information.

On the other hand, think about the case of Jeremy Morgan. He, too, was resistant to PEF monitoring. With the support of his parents, we were able to encourage Jeremy to monitor PEF readings. Although at first he found this to be an intrusion on his daily activities, once the habit was established he found it offered him additional freedom. He is better able to self-manage his disease, and the result has been a significant decrease in his need for medication during the time he spends with his peers.

Change in Patient Status

Although the Expert Panel Report 2 suggests four classifications for asthma, it is not unusual for a patient to vary between classes. Consider the case of Mary Franklin, the college student. In her hometown, she was a patient with mild-intermittent asthma, relying solely on rescue medication and trigger avoidance to successfully manage her disease. The change in environment increased her symptoms and her reliance on rescue medications. The affect of her new environment may have been minimal (a coincidence) or significant (causal). Mary required an increase in medication and intensive education to support this change in her asthma status.

Receipt of Updated or More Complete Patient Information

As discussed in unit 7 of this module, complete patient information seldom reaches pharmacists in ambulatory care practice sites. New information must be incorporated into the treatment plan as it becomes available to you.

Think again about Mary Franklin. She was started on zileuton. She was doing well with her symptoms and her PEF results were good. Lab data then indicated a rise in ALT. This information necessitated a change in Mary's regimen.

New drugs are continually released and new information regarding current therapies becomes available. All of this information must be reworked into the patient's current treatment plan. New information about the effect of inhaled corticosteroids on growth or on cataract development alters the type of monitoring that is done in some patients.

Possible Changes to the Therapy Regimen

There are three changes you can make to a patient's therapy regimen:
- add a new therapy,
- delete a current therapy, or
- modify the current therapy.

All of these changes come about as a result of the evaluation of clearly defined goals and expected outcomes. Without a clear direction for therapy, it is difficult to determine which of these three choices might be best for a patient. The pharmacist in the ambulatory care environment should be sure that the goal of therapy and the expected outcome is clear to each member of the health care team, including the patient.

Adding New Therapy

There are many reasons why a patient with asthma might not be meeting his or her goals of symptom control and infrequent exacerbations. Again, think about Mary Franklin. The change in her status necessitated the addition of new medications when we first encountered her. She still requires a rescue medication; therefore, we are not discontinuing anything from her current regimen. Following the Expert Panel Report 2 guidelines for step therapy, there may be several combinations of medications that will be useful for managing the patient with asthma.

Another example is newly diagnosed 4-year-old Sarah Jacobs. She was successfully treated with Tilade and albuterol until she was exposed to an upper respiratory virus at day care. She experienced an exacerbation requiring oral prednisone for 5 days to bring her symptoms under control. Starting Sarah on the oral prednisone illustrates that a new medication can be added on a short-term basis.

Deleting a Current Therapy

Identifying and communicating goals for your patient will help you determine whether discontinuation is warranted for any particular medication. General goals of pharmacotherapy for patients with asthma include:
- to improve symptoms,
- to minimize exacerbations,
- to incur minimal adverse effects, and
- to facilitate adherence.

Pharmacotherapy that does not achieve these goals must be discontinued. Continuation of medication that has failed a treatment goal is not uncommon in the ambulatory environment. The tendency is to simply add medication rather than subtracting it. The ambulatory care pharmacist can play a pivotal role in ensuring that medication that has not met a goal is discontinued.

In this module, we have discontinued therapy in the patients we have worked with for several of these reasons. Mary Franklin had an adverse effect from her zileuton; Jeremy Morgan was unable to meet adherence goals for his Azmacort regimen, and it was discontinued.

Modifying the Current Therapy Regimen

Unit 21 of the *Core Module* reviews reasons for modifying a patient's therapy regimen. These include:
- development of drug toxicity or adverse events,
- a change in patient status,
- a drug dosage that is not maximized,
- patient nonadherence,
- bioavailability or pharmacokinetic issues, and
- an endpoint that is not met.

Patients empowered with action plans can make modifications to their therapy by following recommendations on their action plans to step up or step down therapy. Patients should be encouraged to record all these modifications and bring the record to each visit so that you can incorporate the information into your patient record.

Changes in Educational Goals and Plans

Factors that might contribute to your decision to alter your educational plan for an ambulatory care patient with asthma include:
- a change in therapy,
- a change in patient status, and
- stabilization of the patient on current therapy.

Change in Therapy

Changes made to a patient's therapy require that additional education be provided. The reason or reasons for the change must be clear to the patient, as well as the goal for this therapy and any additional monitoring that will be done. Remember that the patient will need to carry out the bulk of the plan; his or her understanding of the need for the change and the expected outcome will be vital to achievement of the goal.

Change in Patient Status

Changes in patient status influence the educational plan. A patient's status incorporates not only physical but emotional health as well. Recall Molly, who was introduced in unit 7. We had an intensive education plan designed for her. However, we discovered that her needs at this time are for emotional and family support. Our educational plan is stepped down for the time being.

Stabilization of Patient on Current Therapy

A patient who has reached the desired endpoints and is well controlled needs less frequent educational interventions. It is important to review inhaler technique periodically because it is easy for patients to develop bad habits over time. For example, you may change your educational plan to a yearly from a quarterly review once the patient has reached the desired educational and treatment goals.

Modifying a Pharmacist's Care Plan for Ambulatory Care Patients with Asthma— Case Study

Now that we have reviewed the principles of redesigning a care plan, we will practice making and recording decisions concerning your APCP, monitoring parameters, and therapy.

Review each of Jeremy Morgan's pharmacotherapeutic and related health care goals from the APCP and AMW (**Appendix A**). Based on these documents, determine which modifications, if any, are needed.

Goal #1

First, we wanted to minimize Jeremy's symptoms and optimize his therapy regimen. Monitoring parameters for this goal include assessment of frequency and severity of symptoms and PEF monitoring. The therapeutic interventions included discontinuing the nebulizer solution, starting Serevent at bedtime, and altering the inhaled corticosteroid regimen. Jeremy has progressed towards the desired goal. Nighttime symptoms are currently under control. With the start of Jeremy's participation in cross-country track, we have noted a dip in the evening PEF readings. Based on this information, we need to increase his corticosteroid dose, consider a leukotriene inhibitor, or increase his Serevent to twice a day. We will discuss the options with Jeremy and his mother and determine which choice is preferable.

Goal #2

Our second goal was optimizing education and medication administration. Recall that Jeremy and his mother had reservations about the use of inhaled corticosteroids. Our educational interventions have been successful in alleviating these fears. PEF readings, refill history, and symptom diary have all been completed successfully.

Goal #3

Our third goal was related to Jeremy's experimentation with alcohol and tobacco. We have been unsuccessful at getting Jeremy to share this information with his parents. Although the encounters are less frequent, his experimentation continues, possibly driven by peer pressure. We need to continue to include education directed at recreational drug use in Jeremy's overall education plan.

Goal #4

The fourth goal for Jeremy was to have him do daily PEF monitoring. Although intensive educational intervention was initially necessary to encourage this, Jeremy has now found his ability to monitor and alter his own therapy fulfilling. He realizes the value of this information and the results have lessened his need for medication at school.

Goal #5

The fifth goal for Jeremy was the recognition of his symptoms and an understanding of their severity. The PEF monitoring has helped Jeremy identify his symptoms. We need to continue to monitor his symptom diary to ensure that he continues to recognize his own symptoms as he grows older.

Goal #6

The sixth goal for Jeremy was to discontinue Echinacea. It took significant educational effort to encourage Jeremy's mother to understand that Echinacea has not been shown to be effective for long-term use. She is very interested in alternative therapy. We had to modify Goal #6 to support intermittent use during periods when Jeremy experiences exacerbations or illnesses.

Goal #7

Corticosteroid misconceptions and Jeremy's nonadherence to his corticosteroid therapy regimen were addressed with education and modification to the regimen. Subsequent refills have been consistent with appropriate use.

You can turn to **Appendix B** to see how the pharmacist amended the APCP and AMW as a result of these changes.

Practice Example

Turn to the APCP and AMW for Sarah Jacobs in **Appendix C**. Review your decisions on the achievement of each pharmacotherapeutic and related health goals based on available data. Determine any necessary changes on the APCP. Following the same thought processes as those just used for Jeremy Morgan, make changes to the AMW and APCP for Sarah. Record these changes on the AMW and APCP. Compare your changes with those recorded in **Appendix D**.

Goal #1: Control of Symptoms

Our first goal for Sarah is control of her symptoms. She was initiated on Tilade 2 puffs four times daily and albuterol for rescue therapy. There has been significant confusion about Sarah's medication schedule. She is only in daycare on the weeks she is at her mother's, and the guardians at daycare often forget her dosing at the beginning of the week. Her parents also are confused about the dosing schedule, and it has been difficult for you to evaluate adherence by refill history because only Sarah's mother gets the corticosteroid inhaler filled at your pharmacy. Sarah's father has been using multiple pharmacies to obtain medication. Sarah's technique has declined with time. On questioning, she indicates that the drug tastes "funny" and so she doesn't want to take so much of it. Clearly, the initial recommended regimen needs to be modified. You recommend discontinuing the Tilade and initiating AeroBid, which can be used twice a day. You will need to provide education about the new therapy. Communication with the daycare and with both parents will be necessary. The value of the symptom diary for recording not only symptoms but also medication administration should be emphasized.

Goal #2: Education

Sarah and her parents continue to need additional education regarding asthma and the therapy that is used to treat it. Although they respond appropriately when questioned about triggers and disease course, they have not been successful at incorporating this information into daily decisions.

Goal #3: Influenza Vaccine

Sarah received the influenza vaccine in the fall. We will leave it on the form as it is a yearly vaccination.

Summary

A systematic approach to the evaluation of the implementation of a pharmacist's care plan for an ambulatory care patient with asthma is essential to the redesign of a care plan that meets the patient's needs. The APCP can be altered by changing the patient's pharmacotherapeutic and related health care goals, regimen, monitoring plan, or any combination of these. The pharmacist must be aware of a patient as a complex individual and recognize that any change can cause additional issues to arise.

Reference

1. National Heart, Lung, and Blood Institute. Expert Panel Report 2: Guidelines for the Diagnosis and Management of Asthma. July 1997.

Self-Study Questions

Objective
Determine whether a change in pharmacotherapeutic and health care goals, regimen, or monitoring plan is required in the treatment of ambulatory care patients with asthma.

Review the information for Marie Cowling (**Appendix E**).

1. Decide if a change is needed in the goals we have established for Marie.

2. Decide if a change is needed in the AMW that has been established for Marie.

3. Decide if a change is needed in the APCP that we have developed for Marie.

Objective
Modify a pharmacist's care plan for ambulatory care patients with asthma as necessary based on the achievement of pharmacotherapeutic and related health care goals.

Refer to the case of Marie Cowling, Appendix E.

4. Describe how you will alter your AMW to monitor Marie's progress without PEF readings.

Self-Study Answers

1. Marie will not perform peak flow monitoring. We will need to remove it from our goals and rely on her symptom diary to assess asthma control.

2. We will need to remove the review of PEF readings from the AMW.

3. We need to remove the goal for PEF monitoring.

4. The AMW will need to reflect the importance of the symptom diary. This will be our only tool outside of urgent care visits to evaluate Marie's response to therapy recommendations or the need to modify current therapy.

Ambulatory Pharmacist's Care Plan

Patient __Jeremy Morgan__   Pharmacist __Jennifer Loudon__   Date __March 10, 1999__

DATE IDENTIFIED	PROBLEM (TPL)	PHARMACOTHERAPEUTIC AND RELATED HEALTH CARE GOAL	RECOMMENDATIONS FOR THERAPY	MONITORING PARAMETER(S)	DESIRED ENDPOINT(S)	MONITORING FREQUENCY
3/99	overuse of Albuterol	minimize symptoms optimize therapeutic regimen	D/C Neb solution Institute Serevent 2 puffs @ HS	Frequency & severity of nighttime sx; monitor PEF	PEF >80% No morning dip in PEF; No nighttime symptoms	Each visit
	intermittent refill record Azmacort	optimize education & medication administration	Δ to 1 puff BID Pulmicort	PEF Refill hx symptom diary	Normal PEF No exacerbations adherence	Each visit
	cigarette & Alcohol use	protect confidentiality while educating about risks	Education	Patient report	No exposure	Each visit
	self-monitoring not done	Add peak flow monitoring	Daily PEF & Diary	Diary evaluation	Daily monitor	Each visit
	poor symptom recognition	Educate about symptoms	Education	Patient report	Recognition of symptoms	Each visit
	Echinacea use for prolonged time	Discontinue Echinacea	Discontinue	Patient/parent report	D/C	Each visit
	Influenza vaccine: Not vaccinated	Vaccinate yearly	Vaccinate in the fall	Patient records	vaccination	Every fall
	Misconceptions about corticosteroids	Provide Education	Education	Patient report adherence	adherence	Each visit

© 2000, American Society of Health-System Pharmacists, Inc. All rights reserved.

PHARMACIST'S CARE PLAN AMBULATORY MONITORING WORKSHEET (AMW)

Patient: Jeremy Morgan
Pharmacist: Jennifer Loudon
Date: 3/10/99

Pharmaco-therapeutic Goal	Monitoring Parameter	Desired Endpoint	Monitoring Frequency	Date 3/10/99	4/3	5/5	6/20	7/30	9/20
Improve asthma control	Symptom Diary	↓ freq. of sx	q month		↑Sx ✓	↑Sx ✓	↓Sx ✓	↓Sx ✓	↓Sx ✓
	Beta-adrenergic agonist use (refill hx)	<1 canister per month	q month		OK	OK	OK	OK	OK
	Pulmicort use (refill hx)	No gaps in refill	q month		OK	OK	OK	OK	OK
	Nighttime Sx	None	(patient) Daily		←	ER visit ↑	→	→	↑
Monitoring of peak flow	Morning PEF	Daily ✓'s	(patient) Daily		420	400	420	420	420
	Influenza vaccine	Given	q fall		—	—	—	—	done
Education	Patient knowledge	Understanding	q visit		✓	✓	✓	✓	✓
	Inhaler technique	Appropriate	q visit		✓	✓	✓	✓	✓
Monitoring	Evening PEF	Daily ✓'s	q visit			started ✓'s △	440 △	450 △	390 →
cigarette & alcohol education	Patient/parent report	0 exposures	q visit		2-3	5	1	2	2
d/c echinacea	Patient/parent report	D/C	q visit		Patient is still using				

© 2000, American Society of Health-System Pharmacists, Inc. All rights reserved.

Ambulatory Pharmacist's Care Plan

Patient: Jeremy Morgan Pharmacist: Jennifer Loudon Date: December 1999

Revised

DATE IDENTIFIED	PROBLEM (TPL)	PHARMACOTHERAPEUTIC AND RELATED HEALTH CARE GOAL	RECOMMENDATIONS FOR THERAPY	MONITORING PARAMETER(S)	DESIRED ENDPOINT(S)	MONITORING FREQUENCY
3/99	Ongoing asthma management	Symptom management self-management optimal therapeutic regime	↑ Serevent to 2 puffs BID or ↑ Pulmicort to 2 puffs BID	Morning & Evening PEF symptoms (Diary) Continue √'ing refill Hx	No PEF Dip in evening No symptoms	Each visit
3/99	Ongoing self-monitoring	Daily peak flow monitoring; morning & evening	continue monitoring & recording in diary	Morning & evening PEF	PEF >80% √'d daily	Each visit
3/99	Ongoing cigarette & alcohol use	continue to protect confidentiality & educate	education	patient report	No exposure-discuss w/ parents (Jeremy to discuss)	Each visit
12/99	Echinacea use	Periodic use of Echinacea for immune-stimulation	No continuous use-periodic use when symptoms ↑	patient/parent report	No continuous use- No more than 6 week @ a time	Each visit
3/99	Influenza vaccine	Yearly influenza vaccine	vaccinate every fall	Pt. records	vaccination	Each fall
3/99	ongoing education	Patient/parent understanding	Continued education	Pt. report inhaler technique	Pt. understanding Inhaler technique appropriate	Each visit

PHARMACIST'S CARE PLAN AMBULATORY MONITORING WORKSHEET (AMW)

Patient __Jeremy Morgan__ Pharmacist __Jennifer Loudon__
   __Revised__ Date __December 1999__

Pharmaco-therapeutic Goal	Monitoring Parameter	Desired Endpoint	Monitoring Frequency	Date											
ongoing asthma management & self-monitoring	morning & evening PEF	No dips in A.M. or P.M.	q visit												
	symptom diary	No ↑ exacerb. % treatment	q visit												
	Refill Hx Pulmicort	No gaps or overuse	q visit												
	Refill Hx Albuterol	<1 canister q month	q visit												
daily PEF monitoring	PEF record	daily √'s PEF >80%	q visit												
cigarette & alcohol ed.	patient report	0 exposures parents told	q visit												
Periodic echinacea use	patient/parent report	No more than 6 wks of therapy	q visit												
vaccination Influenza	Records-Influenza vaccine	vaccinated	q Fall												
education	patient/parent understanding	understanding	q visit												
↓	Inhaler technique	appropriate	q visit												

© 2000, American Society of Health-System Pharmacists, Inc. All rights reserved.

Ambulatory Pharmacist's Care Plan

Patient: Sarah Jacobs Pharmacist: Bill Jelen Date: 4-99

DATE IDENTIFIED	PROBLEM (TPL)	PHARMACOTHERAPEUTIC AND RELATED HEALTH CARE GOAL	RECOMMENDATIONS FOR THERAPY	MONITORING PARAMETER(S)	DESIRED ENDPOINT(S)	MONITORING FREQUENCY
4/6/99	New diagnosis asthma—associated w/viral illness	control of sxs	Tilade 2 puffs qid Albuterol qid prn	symptoms exacerbations refill hx gaps in refill	minimal sxs no exacerbations, appropriate refills	q visit q refill
4/6	Basic asthma education needed	Education	Set up education plan—will need to include both parents	✓ patient/parent understanding	patient/parent understanding pathophys & meds	q visit
4/6	No flu vaccine	vaccination in fall	schedule in fall	✓ if received	vaccinated	q fall

* 12/99 received oral prednisone × 5 days exac resulted from exp to resp virus, failure to adhere to tx regimen

© 2000, American Society of Health-System Pharmacists, Inc. All rights reserved.

PHARMACIST'S CARE PLAN AMBULATORY MONITORING WORKSHEET (AMW)

Patient __Sarah Jacobs__　　　　　　　　　　　　　　　　　　　　Pharmacist __Bill Jelen__
　　　　　　　　　　　　　　　　　　　　　　　　　　　　　　　　　　Date __4-6-99__

Pharmaco-therapeutic Goal	Monitoring Parameter	Desired Endpoint	Monitoring Frequency	Date 4/6	5/20	6/30	9/30	11/20	11/20	2/22
Asthma control	Symptom diary	No symptoms	q visit		OK ✓	OK ✓	OK ✓	OK ✓	↑2 ER visits ↑'d sxs	↑'d sxs
Med Adherence	Albuterol refill hx	<1 cannister per month	q visit		✓	*	*	*	*	*
Med Adherence	Tilade refill hx	No gaps in refill	q visit		✓	*	*	*	*	*
Technique	Patient inhaler demonstration	Appr. technique	q visit		some difficulty	improved	good	not as good	poor	poor
Education	Patient/parent understanding	understanding	q visit		needs help	improved	improved	good	good	good
Vaccine	Influenza vaccine	vaccine q fall	q fall		—	—	vaccinated	—	—	—

*cannot evaluate due to medications filled @ multiple pharmacies
Patient reports poor taste in mouth not wanting "to take it all"!

© 2000, American Society of Health-System Pharmacists, Inc. All rights reserved.

Ambulatory Pharmacist's Care Plan

Patient: Sarah Jacobs Pharmacist: Bill Jelen Date: 4-99

DATE IDENTIFIED	PROBLEM (TPL)	PHARMACOTHERAPEUTIC AND RELATED HEALTH CARE GOAL	RECOMMENDATIONS FOR THERAPY	MONITORING PARAMETER(S)	DESIRED ENDPOINT(S)	MONITORING FREQUENCY
4/6/99	New diagnosis asthma-associated w/viral illness	control of sxs	Tilade 2 puffs qid Albuterol qid prn *(modified see below)*	symptoms exacerbations refill hx gaps in refill	minimal sxs no exacerbations, appropriate refills	q visit q refill
4/6	Basic asthma education needed	Education	Set up education plan—will need to include both parents	✓ patient/parent understanding	patient/parent understanding pathophys & meds	q visit
4/6 reaffirm 2/22	No flu vaccine	vaccination in fall	schedule in fall	✓ if received	vaccinated	q fall
2/22/00	↑'d symptoms poor adherence	control of symptoms	DC Tilade continue Albuterol Start Aerobid 1 puff-bid	symptoms exacerbations	minimal sxs no exacerbations	q visit
2/22/00	Basic education	Education-patient/parent able to make daily decisions	continue to emphasize Mom to attend support group	✓ patient/parent understanding ✓ symptom diary	understanding & able to incorporate into daily decisions	q visit

* 12/99 received oral prednesone ⓧ 5 days exac resulted from exp to resp virus, failure to adhere to tx regimen

PHARMACIST'S CARE PLAN AMBULATORY MONITORING WORKSHEET (AMW)

Patient Sarah Jacobs
Revised 2/22

Pharmacist Bill Jelen
Date 2/22/00

Pharmaco-therapeutic Goal	Monitoring Parameter	Desired Endpoint	Monitoring Frequency	Date 2/22													
Asthma control	Symptom Diary	No sxs	q visit														
Med Adherence	Albuterol use	minimal	√ diary q visit														
Med Adherence	Aerobid	adherent	√ diary q visit														
Technique	Patient inhaler demonstration	appr. technique	q visit														
Education	Patient/parent understanding	understanding	q visit														
Vaccine	Influenza vaccine	vaccine q fall	q fall														
No Side Effects	Patient report	No adverse effects	q visit														

© 2000, American Society of Health-System Pharmacists, Inc. All rights reserved.

Ambulatory Pharmacist's Care Plan

Patient: Marie Cowling Pharmacist: Jim Bellows Date: July 8, 1999

DATE IDENTIFIED	PROBLEM (TPL)	PHARMACOTHERAPEUTIC AND RELATED HEALTH CARE GOAL	RECOMMENDATIONS FOR THERAPY	MONITORING PARAMETER(S)	DESIRED ENDPOINT(S)	MONITORING FREQUENCY
7/8/99	Overuse of Beta-adrenergic agonist	Use Beta-adrenergic agonist appropriately & have good disease control	Add Aerobid 2 puffs BID ↓ use of Maxair use PRN	Patient report Refill hx	appropriate use of beta-adrenergic agonist	each visit
	No local health care provider	Establish relationship with local physician	Refer to Joan Owens-social worker for MD Referral	√ c̄ patient	patient establishes relationship with local provider	N/A
	No PEF monitoring	PEF monitoring	Daily PEF to establish personal best then periodic assessment	Patient diary	patient able to self-manage symptoms	each visit
	Possible drug-disease interaction	No drug-disease interaction	DC ibuprofen use Tylenol for osteoarthritis pain	Patient report	relief from arthritis	each visit
	improved disease control	Asthma control	patient education Identify trigger patient will need symptom diary	Patient report ↑ Qa-walking c/o sx	symptom control	each visit
↓	Arthritis	control of arthritis symptoms	DC ibuprofen use Tylenol for osteoarthritis pain	Patient report	Relief from arthritis	each visit

PHARMACIST'S CARE PLAN AMBULATORY MONITORING WORKSHEET (AMW)

Patient __Marie Cowling__ Pharmacist __Jim Bellows__
Date __July 1999__

Pharmaco-therapeutic Goal	Monitoring Parameter	Desired Endpoint	Monitoring Frequency	Date 7/8/99	8/15	9/28	11/20									
Symptom control	Patient diary	minimal symptoms	pt √'s daily diary √ 2 visit		↑ sx	↑ sx	↑ sx									
PEF monitoring	Patient diary	establish personal best	next visit		* Re-fuses	* Re-fuses	* Re-fuses									
Arthritis control	Patient report	free of symptoms	each visit		↑ sx	↑ sx	↑ sx									
medication use	Maxair use	<1 canister per month	each visit		2 canisters	2 canisters	2 canisters									
↓	AeroBID use	No gaps	each visit		gap in fill	gap in fill	ok									

*Pt refuses to monitor PEF

Ambulatory Pharmacist's Care Plan

Patient: Mary Franklin   Pharmacist: Cheryl Marks   Date: 9/20/99

DATE IDENTIFIED	PROBLEM (TPL)	PHARMACOTHERAPEUTIC AND RELATED HEALTH CARE GOAL	RECOMMENDATIONS FOR THERAPY	MONITORING PARAMETER(S)	DESIRED ENDPOINT(S)	MONITORING FREQUENCY
9/20/99	Overuse of Beta-Adrenergic agonist	Appropriate use & maintain disease control	Evaluate for addition of inhaled corticosteroid	symptom report, symptom diary	Appropriate use	Each visit
	No local provider	Local health care provider identified	Given names of physicians	Patient report	Local health care provider	Next visit
	No PEF monitoring	Daily PEF reading to establish personal best & periodic	Education	Diary	Periodic PEF monitoring	Each visit
	Baseline Education	Understanding of medication use and disease	Education	Patient report	Understanding	Each visit
	Asthma poorly controlled	Education medication management	Add inhaled corticosteroid AeroBid 3 puffs BID	symptoms, PEF, LFTs, refill history	Reduce exacerbations	Each visit, LFTs per protocol
			Rec. zileuton 20mg BID			

* 11/15 Begin zileuton

2/00 Zileuton dc'd ↑Aerobid to 5 puffs BID

© 2000, American Society of Health-System Pharmacists, Inc. All rights reserved.

PHARMACIST'S CARE PLAN AMBULATORY MONITORING WORKSHEET (AMW)

Patient: Mary Franklin
Pharmacist: Patti Belle
Date: Sept. 1999

Pharmacotherapeutic Goal	Monitoring Parameter	Desired Endpoint	Monitoring Frequency	10/2	11/15	12/5	1/15	2/15	3/15	5/15	7/15	9/10
Symptom control	pt diary-symptoms	↓ frequency	q visit		←	↓	OK	OK	OK	OK	↓	
	Beta-adrenergic agonist (refill hx)	<1 canister/month	q visit		2 canisters	↓	↓	↓	↓	↓	2 canisters	2 canisters *
	AeroBid use (refill hx)	No gaps	q visit		gap	OK	OK	OK	OK	OK	1 gap	gap
	Nighttime sx	No sx	q visit		←	None	None	None	None	None	←	←
Monitoring	Morning PEF	daily √'s	q visit		not done	√ 325	√ 350	√ 350	√ 360	√ 380	290	305
	Influenza vaccine	vaccine	q fall	done								vaccine
Knowledge	pt knowledge	understanding	q visit		improving	OK	OK	OK	OK	OK	OK	OK
	Inhaler technique	appropriate	q visit		good	good	good	good	good	good	good	good
Adverse effects	ALT	0-35 units/L	q month MD office		5	15	30	60	20	10		

*Pt self-DC'D 2° to concerns about recurrent vaginal candidiasis